Crafts
in Therapy
and Rehabilitation

Margaret Drake, PhD, OTR/L, A.T.R.

University of Alabama at Birmingham

SLACK Incorporated, 6900 Grove Road, Thorofare, NJ 08086-9447

Illustrations by Cynthia Bishop and Bob Hochgertel, based on original sketches by the author.

Drake, Margaret.
    Crafts in therapy and rehabilitation.

    Includes bibliographical references and index.
    1. Handicraft—Therapeutic use.   2. Occupational therapy.   I. Title.
[DNLM: 1. Handicapped.   2. Occupational therapy—methods.   3. Psychomotor
Performance.   4. Rehabilitation, Vocational. WB 555 D762c]
RM735.7.H35D73 1992   615.8′515   89-42919
ISBN 1-55642-118-4 (pbk.)

Printed in the United States of America

Published by: SLACK Incorporated
                6900 Grove Road
                Thorofare, NJ 08086-9447

Last digit is print number: 10   9   8   7   6   5   4

To my stepmother, Jessie N. Williams,
who showed me the possibilities of crafts.

Contents

Acknowledgments   vii
Preface   ix

Part I   Introduction to Crafts   1
Chapter 1   Therapeutic Use of Crafts: What are Crafts?   3
Chapter 2   Frames of Reference: Implications for the
              Use of Crafts   9
Chapter 3   Choosing an Activity and Assessing
              Therapeutic Application   17
Chapter 4   Analyzing and Grading Activities   21
Chapter 5   Shall I Use a Kit or Start from Scratch?   27

Part II   The Major Crafts Used Clinically by Therapists   31
Chapter 6   Woodworking   33
Chapter 7   Leatherwork   47
Chapter 8   Needlework   63
Chapter 9   Copper Tooling and Metal Craft   71
Chapter 10 Mosaics   81
Chapter 11 Ceramics   91
Chapter 12 Weaving, Latchook, Macramé and Other
              Fiber Crafts   111

**Part III Nontraditional Crafts and Minor Media
            Activities Used Clinically in Therapy   121**
Chapter 13 Paper Crafts   123
Chapter 14 Cooking as a Craft   137
Chapter 15 Computer Art as a Craft   149
Chapter 16 Art Techniques: Drawing and Painting   157
Chapter 17 Other Frequently Used Crafts   169
Chapter 18 Miscellaneous Creative Media   179

Appendices   187
Appendix I   Vendors of Materials Described in this Text   189
Appendix II   Annotated Bibliography   191
Appendix III Completed Activity Analysis   199

Index   207

Acknowledgments

Many others have assisted in the creation of this book. My secretaries, Venita Edwards and Vicki Cross, have been unfailingly cheerful, helpful and tolerant. My colleagues in the Division of Occupational Therapy at The University of Alabama at Birmingham, Carroline Amari, OTR/L; Louise Thibodaux, OTR/L; Patty Barnett, COTA/L; Angela Griffin, OTR/L; Jan Rowe, OTR/L; Richard Maynard, OTR/L; and Larry Zachow, OTR/L have contributed proofreading, suggestions and encouragement. Alabama therapists Elsie McKibbin, OTR/L; Tina Scarborough, OTR/L; Barbara Edwards, OTR/L; Jeannie Cottingham, OTR/L; Mimi Fowlkes, OTR/L; Jane McGee, OTR/L; Roy Donaldson, OTR/L; Christine Washington, OTR/L; Connie Dasher, OTR/L; Albertha Lyas; Ron Jenke, OTR/L; Lee Sumner, OTR/L; Amanda Neighbors, COTA/L; David Garst, OTR/L; Denise Murray, OTR/L. Kim Lawrence and Amelia Spencer have assisted with ideas, suggestions and encouragement. May Robertson made suggestions in the chapter on ceramics. Nutritionist Carol Craig assisted with resources for the cooking chapter. Judy White, Benjamin White, Ali Solymani, Jesus Mercado and Christopher Lynch contributed ideas and proofreading on the computer chapter. I am grateful to all these friends and colleagues and to the professional reviewers.

—Margaret Drake

Preface

This book explains the value of crafts in occupational therapy treatment for students, interns and occupational therapy clinicians. It adopts a historical–anthropological approach to development of crafts, examining the human experience and describing global patterns as well as what is unique to a particular cultural group. Each chapter is prefaced by a brief historical and anthropological look at the craft described. The prevalence of the current use of each craft is discussed. Because the first step in occupational therapy treatment is screening and evaluation, the text tells which formal occupational therapy evaluations are available that use the various crafts. Occupational therapists need to know the various crafts in order to perform these evaluations.

Examples of crafts that can be used with today's short-stay patients are presented in a step-by-step format. Therapeutic applications as well as contraindications are discussed for physical dysfunction, mental health, pediatrics and geriatrics. Most chapters present a case study that demonstrates a clinical context in which the craft has been used successfully. The people appearing in the case studies represent the ethnic diversity, different age ranges and variety of diagnoses that occupational therapists find in their caseloads. Discussion questions are intended to be thought provoking and to help elicit problem-solving capabilities. Because today's therapists have so much to read, this text is written in a simple yet lively fashion. The addresses and telephone numbers of craft suppliers are provided in Appendix I, as students and therapists often need this information. An annotated reference list provides bibliographic information on books related to each of the craft categories described in this book. In short, this text is intended to help students, interns and occupational therapists use crafts in patient treatment.

Part

I

Introduction to Crafts

1
Therapeutic Use of Crafts: What are Crafts?

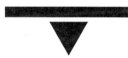

craft (kraft) an occupation requiring special skill;
especially any of the manual arts[1]

Why is the use of crafts in occupational therapy a topic to be explored? In this time of shortened hospital stays and limited resources for supply and equipment budgets, therapists are forced to streamline their treatment procedures. Information technology products, such as computers and videos, which have thrust us into the current information age have also carried us away from and obscured the usefulness of one of our very helpful modalities of occupational therapy treatment, crafts. We have moved toward more frequent use of electronic media in patient treatment, such as computers and videos, and while that may not diminish the emphasis on what we do with our hands and bodies, the reality is that so little time is available for treatment of patients that therapists must choose among treatment modalities and many choose computers.

Additionally, in a work-oriented culture like ours, crafts have come to symbolize a leisure time activity rather than *real* work. As medical diagnostic and treatment technology has mushroomed, occupational therapy has been forced to appear more scientific. Somehow, crafts do not seem scientific. Even as early as 1924, the Boston School of Occupational Therapy defined our profession with emphasis on the scientific and measurable use of activities to achieve reduction of dysfunction.[2] However, as in medicine, where physicians are beginning to realize that quality time spent interviewing/listening to a patient produces as much information as more expensive tests and procedures, occupational therapists are realizing that our traditional methods also produce valuable results.

More than half of all occupational therapy clinics treating pediatric, geriatric, physical dysfunction and mentally ill patients continue to use basic crafts such as leatherwork and needlework in treatment.[3] Certainly, as many therapists use crafts as use splints.

As our literature has developed over the last two decades, the word crafts has been almost obliterated from the professional vocabulary. Rather than say craft group or craft session, we say *task group*[4] or *dyadic interaction skills group*.[5] Task group is a term that came into use in the late 1960s.[6] Early photographs in *A Functional Approach to Group Work in Occupational Therapy* by Howe and Schwartzberg[7] have titles of task group and project group when what they were doing were crafts. Textbooks from the last 50 years show how the terminology related to crafts has changed. This is described in more detail later in this chapter. We need to revalue for ourselves the usefulness of craft media in treatment.[8]

Crafts in particular help patients realize that through the process of taking raw materials or minimally prepared substances and processing, assembling and forming them, that the patients can do the same with their life. Crafts are a microcosm of life—one receives basic raw materials, and through a series of efforts, waiting periods and guidance one lives a life—one creates a craft product. Crafts are a teaching example of how to put it all together. This concept makes crafts valuable therapeutic media for the modern clinical setting with short-term hospital stays.

As we learn more about brain lateralization and localized specialization, we know that crafts are able to naturally use the spatial and intuitive functions of the nondominant side of the brain.[9-12] We, as a profession, have intuitively understood that crafts help use and rehabilitate brain functions but we did not know why.

Now this information is gradually being authenticated through research.[13,14] There is scientific evidence to show why crafts perform rehabilitative functions that exercise or other activities do less efficiently.[15] While use of crafts cannot do everything, they are important and valid treatment media. We do not want to go back to a time when there were only a few treatment modalities with crafts being the main one. It is important to keep crafts as one of many treatment alternatives.

A look at the indices and tables of content of the profession's textbooks over the years gives a little insight into how crafts were viewed. The very first edition of *Occupational Therapy* by Willard and Spackman[16] lists seven crafts in the index under activities. The word handicrafts was used to define another 18 items. All but one of the 15 photographs show a craft in progress. The second edition, *Principles of Occupational Therapy*[17] does not use the word crafts in the index, but under activities, lists 14 separate crafts. The title of a section of the chapter *Activities in Occupational Therapy* is *Handicrafts*.

Most of the *Activities Suggested to Provide Treatment* in the third edition[18] are crafts; however, a glance through the table of contents and index gives almost no hint that crafts are a major activity. By the fourth edition,[19] under activities in the index, no crafts are named, but when one turns to the page for *Activities for Restoration of Function* most of the activities listed are indeed crafts. In the fifth edition[20] one must search to find an allusion to crafts. Euphemisms such as *functional activities* or *avocational activities* are used instead. The sixth edition[21] contains one paragraph entitled *To Use Crafts or Not to Use Crafts?* This 1983 text lists leatherlacing, woodworking and crafts with *therapeutic use* in the index. The seventh edition[22] reflects the increased use of computer technology with 11 index listings for computers and one for *crafts as therapy*. Throughout the chapter on historical perspectives, attitudes toward crafts by the profession's leaders are mentioned.

Another text, *Prescribing Occupational Therapy*,[23] by physician Dr. William Dunton, emphasizes the prescription from physicians for occupational therapy treatment. This book tells how the therapist may be in a better position than the physician to choose activities. A ten-page section gives *Suggestions for the Use of Crafts in Functional Restoration* plus a 15-item guide for selection that emphasizes craft quality and usefulness.

Many books currently being used that one would assume would mention crafts, do not list them in the index.[2,24-28] On the other hand, other texts reflect the value of crafts and do list them.[7,29,32] This exemplifies the ambivalence felt by many occupational therapists to these modalities, which are used in many clinics. Barris, Kielhofner and Watts[32] attribute the diminishing discussion of crafts in occupational therapy "to the general devaluation of handmade objects in American culture."

In a 1986 study[3] and a 1988 study in which Barris collaborated, cooking was found to be the most commonly used craft. Therapists answering the surveys worked in physical disabilities, mental health, pediatrics, developmental disabilities, hand clinics, geriatrics and institutions that treat the whole range of disabilities. A 1989 survey with unpublished results from Florida International University[33] on "what crafts are being taught in occupational therapy programs" found a similar ranking in which crafts are used more often: woodworking, leather, needlework, copper tooling, mosaics and ceramics, followed by a number of other crafts. The chapters of this book are organized around this frequency ranking with the more frequently used crafts coming first.

Associations of pottery and weaving with goddess worship have been suggested as evidence that these crafts were invented by women.[34] Many crafts were invented by women to assist them in their primary role as mother and nurturer. Early woodworking and leathercraft for women would have included making cradles and cradleboards to carry babies on their backs while they went to get food or tend animals. We know that in hunter-gatherer cultures, men killed and brought home the game and women prepared the hides[35-39] and sewed them together for clothes, shelter and food containers. With the development of metal, men began to take over some crafts as they developed more efficient weapons and warfare. As patriarchy prevailed, men took over many prestigious crafts such as woodworking and pottery. When the industrial revolution swept away many handicrafts, those that remained, like needlework and china painting, again became the province of women.[35,40] While men continued to dominate woodworking, leathercraft and pottery in western culture, possibly the decline in status for some crafts has to do with their identification with women.

Historically, documentation of crafts in health treatment is sketchy until the late 18th century. Music as treatment is more commonly mentioned among the ancients.[17] In earlier times, as noted above, crafts were undoubtedly a necessity for clothing, food containers, implements and tools. Something so integral to daily life may not have had the healing properties that we attribute to crafts today. However, Rich[37] credits early arts such as weaving and pottery with magical qualities although rituals and taboos among primitive peoples have been given more credit than crafts for producing cures.[41]

Galen, the Greek physician who adopted Rome as his home, did recommend exercise[42] and felt that patients are healed by being occupied;[17] however, he did not specify crafts. The Arabs adopted much of what was good from Greek and Roman medicine. Ibn Jazlah, an Arabic physician in the Middle Ages (AD 500—1500) recommended physical treatment such as baths and exercise.[43] Some tribes of Native Americans, such as the Navaho and Cheyenne, have traditionally used painting and sand painting in healing and medicine.[41] In Europe, during the Middle Ages, enlightened and humane patient treatment for most disorders was eclipsed.

With the development of humane treatment of patients in Europe at the beginning of the 19th century, Phillipe Pinel persuaded tradesmen in Paris to give craft work to his patients in Aisle de Bicetre.[44] Throughout Europe, similar developments in humane treatment followed.

About that same time, Dr. Benjamin Rush, signer of the Declaration of Independence and Father of American Psychiatry, used work and some crafts with his patients at Pennsylvania Hospital in Philadelphia.[17,45] By mid-century, patients' craft work was being advertised for sale in London.[45] Up through the latter part of the 19th century, many mental hospitals developed programs that included occupations, amusements and crafts.

Probably the first professional writing occupational therapists have on crafts in treatment is *Studies in Invalid Occupation*.[46] The author, Susan Tracy, was the first to designate specific crafts for specific needs. From then on, publications in occupational therapy included instructions on how to use crafts to treat patients. The refinement of skills in choosing the best activity for each patient continues. This book further presents the use of crafts in health care for an era in which faster is better and in which competition and quantity production are the emphasized, valued ethic and norm rather than quality, hand-crafted articles.

References

1. Webster's New World Dictionary, 2nd College Edition. (1982).
2. Reed, K.L. & Sanderson, S.R. (1983). *Concepts of Occupational Therapy*, 2nd ed. Baltimore: Williams and Wilkins.
3. Barris, R., Cordero, J. & Christiaansen, R. (1986). Occupational therapist's use of media. *American Journal of Occupational Therapy*, 40 (10): 679-684.
4. Fidler, G.S. (1984). *Design of Rehabilitation Services in Psychiatric Hospital Settings*. Laurel, MD: Ramsco Publishing Co.
5. Arbesman, F., et al. (1984). *Occupational Therapy: Protocols in Mental Health*. Baltimore: Betty Cox Associates.
6. Fidler, G.S. (1969). The task-oriented group as a context for treatment. *American Journal of Occupational Therapy*. 23 (1): 43-48.
7. Howe, M. & Schwartberg, S. (1986). *A Functional Approach to Group Work in Occupational Therapy*. Philadelphia: Lippincott.
8. Fidler, G.S. & Fidler, J.W.A. (1981). From crafts to competence. *American Journal of Occupational Therapy*, 35 (9): 567-573.
9. Miller, L. (1988a). The emotional brain. *Psychology Today*, 22 (2): 34-42.
10. Miller. L. (1988b). Men without passion. *Psychology Today*, 22 (12): 20-22.
11. Ornstein, R.E. (1972). *The Psychology of Consciousness*. San Francisco: W.H. Freeman and Company.
12. Rosenfeld, A.A. (1988). New images, new insights into your brain. *Psychology Today*, 22 (11): 22-24.
13. Corballis, M. & Beals, I. (1983). *The Ambivalent Mind*. Chicago: Nelson-Hall.
14. Herrmann, N. (1988). *The Creative Brain*. Lake Lure, NC: Applied Creative Services.
15. Thibodaux, C.S. & Ludwig, F.M. (1988). Intrinsic movement in product-oriented and non-product-oriented activities. *American Journal of Occupational Therapy*, 42 (3): 169-175.
16. Willard, H.S. & Spackman, C.E. (1947). *Principles of Occupational Therapy*. Philadelphia: Lippincott.
17. Willard, H.S. & Spackman, C.E. (1954). *Principles of Occupational Therapy*, 2nd ed. Philadelphia: Lippincott.
18. Willard, H.S. & Spackman, C.E. (1963). *Occupational Therapy*, 3rd ed. Philadelphia: Lippincott.
19. Willard, H.S. & Spackman, C.E. (1971). *Occupational Therapy*, 4th ed. Philadelphia: Lippincott.
20. Hopkins, H.L. & Smith, H.D. (1978). *Willard and Spackman's Occupational Therapy*, 5th ed. Philadelphia: Lippincott.
21. Hopkins, H.L. & Smith, H.D. (1983). *Willard and Spackman's Occupational Therapy*, 6th ed. Philadelphia: Lippincott.
22. Hopkins, H.L. & Smith, H.D. (1988). *Willard and Spackman's Occupational Therapy*, 7th ed. Philadelphia: Lippincott.
23. Dunton, W.R. (1945). *Prescribing Occupational Therapy*, 2nd ed. Springfield, IL: Charles C. Thomas.

24. Bruce, M.A. & Borg, B. (1987). *Frames of Reference in Occupational Therapy.* Thorofare, NJ: Slack.
25. Cynkin, S. & Robinson, A.M. (1990). *Occupational Therapy and Activities Health: Toward Health Through Activities.* Boston: Little, Brown and Co.
26. Mosey, A.C. (1986). *Psychosocial Components of Occupational Therapy.* New York: Raven Press.
27. Reed, K.L. (1984). *Models of Practice in Occupational Therapy.* Baltimore: Williams and Wilkins.
28. Trombly, C.A. (1983). *Occupational Therapy for Physical Dysfunction,* 2nd ed. Baltimore: Williams and Wilkins.
29. Early, M.B. (1987). *Mental Health Concepts and Technique for the Occupational Therapy Assistant.* New York: Raven Press.
30. Kaplan, K.L. (1988). *Directive Group Therapy: Innovative Mental Health Treatment.* Thorofare, NJ: Slack.
31. Ryan, S., ed. (1986). *The Certified Occupational Therapy Assistant: Roles and Responsibilities.* Thorofare, NJ: Slack.
32. Barris, R., Kielhofner, G & Watts, J. (1988). *Occupational Therapy in Psychosocial Practice.* Thorofare, NJ: Slack.
33. Florida International University. (1989).
34. Eisler, R. (1987). *The Chalice and the Blade.* New York: Harper and Row.
35. Boserup, E. (1970). *Women's Role in Economic Development.* London: George Allen and Unwin.
36. Morgan, E. (1972). *The Descent of Woman.* New York: Stein and Day.
37. Rich, A. (1976). *Of Women Born.* New York: Bantam Books.
38. Sanday, P.R. (1981). *Female Power and Male Dominance: On the Origins of Sexual Inequality.* Cambridge: Cambridge University Press.
39. Whyte, M.K. (1978). *The Status of Women in Preindustrial Societies.* Princeton, NJ: Princeton University Press.
40. Sochen, J. (1974). *Her Story: A Women's View of American History.* New York: Alfred Publishing Co.
41. Achterknecht, E.H. (1971). *Medicine and Ethnology: Elements and Exercises.* Lawrence, KS: The University of Kansas Press.
42. MacKenzie, J. (1979). *The History of Health and Art of Preserving It.* New York: Arno Press.
43. Graziani, J.S. (1980). *Arabic Medicine in the Eleventh Century as Represented in the Works of Ibn Jazlah.* Karachi, Pakistan: Hamard Academy Press.
44. Pinel, P. (1806). *Traite Medico-Philosophique de l'Alienation Mentale.* Paris: J.A. Brosson.
45. Haworth, N.A. & MacDonald, E.M. (1946). *Theory of Occupational Therapy.* Baltimore: Williams and Wilkins.
46. Tracy, S. (1910). *A Manual for Nurses and Attendants: Studies in Invalid Occupations.* Boston: Whitcomb Barrows.

2
Frames of Reference: Implications for the Use of Crafts

Introduction

Frames of reference is a term that has come to mean how a therapist thinks about treatment and why she thinks a treatment will work with her patients in occupational therapy. Each frame of reference is based on a theory. A theory is an idea about why life is like it is, and why things and people work the way they work. "Theory is not static, nor is it ever final."[1] When authors choose different frames of reference to include in their books, each decides which ones have the most important and relevant ideas. Sometimes different names are given to frames of references that appear to be essentially the same. In the interest of simplicity and clarity, only the ones from the American Occupational Therapy Association (AOTA) *Focus-Skills for Assessment and Treatment* workshops[2] and from *Willard and Spackman's Occupational Therapy*[3] have been included in this text.

Theories with a similar theoretical base and view of illness and activity are grouped under one heading. Some writers call them models rather than frames of reference. This can be confusing. The term *frame of reference* is used in this text because it is commonly used by AOTA. Each frame of reference discussed here will include a view of humanity, of illness, of therapies including activities, and, specifically, craft activities.[4-6]

Frames of reference are based on concepts and principles about how to work with particular problems. For example, a person who operated on the principle that all development of morals takes place before the age of six will have a different approach to teen and adult patients than a person who believes in the concept that humans are always learning and growing morally. The first person might strongly believe in incarceration and punishment while the second would believe in providing many learning and growing experiences. The first person might use certain crafts as punishment or might deprive the patient of crafts as punishment. The second person would want to use only crafts that would provide new learning for patients or that could provide altruistic experiences such as making toys for a children's hospital. The principles underlying each approach would greatly affect which crafts were offered, which tools were allowed, where they might be used and almost every other aspect of the decision-making process. Therefore, the frames of reference that give meaning to these concepts and principles become very important to the individual therapist. For this reason, the student needs to evaluate and compare the concepts and principles underlying the frames of reference to follow.

The Neurophysiologic Frame of Reference

Human function is made up of a balance of biochemical and biological processes. The function of each human is expressed in the integration of sensory input and perceptual-motor output. This input-output process constitutes demonstrated behavior. As a result of illness or defects in the brain in the vestibular, proprioceptive, visual and auditory systems, or in processing and integration of sensations in these systems, abnormal behavior may result.

Occupational therapy treatment attempts to reverse this defective integration and processing. Sensory integration often becomes the goal of treatment. It may be achieved by activities that involve gross motor body movements. Heavy work patterns are considered normalizers of neurotransmitter balance in the neural system. Such activities also metabolize stress hormones and reduce abnormal feelings and reactions. Crafts that involve heavy work patterns and postural changes are considered most likely to achieve sensory integration. Sawing, hammering, throwing and mixing can be used to achieve these goals in this frame of reference.[2,3]

The Cognitive Disabilities Frame of Reference

Humans are defined by their cognitive abilities, demonstrated in their ability to speak and use language and to change and preserve material objects. Symbols, words and language are important in assessing cognitive levels and conscious awareness. According to this frame of reference, illness or dysfunction has a natural cause that may be manifested by changes in cognitive levels. This frame of reference assumes that there is a relationship between biologic abnormalities and psychiatric diseases. Mental illness is considered to include impairment in sensorimotor information processing.[7]

One important function of the occupational therapist in the cognitive disabilities frame of reference is to assess a patient's cognitive level according to task performance. In planning treatment, challenging activities slightly beyond the patient's current functional level are avoided. The patient's ability to work with materials may change. The therapist must be attentive to cognitive level changes and provide activities at the appropriate level. The Allen Cognitive Levels (ACL) Test involves leatherlacing. A variety of craft materials and activities is considered appropriate for the different cognitive levels. In the book *Cognitive Disabilities: Expanded Activity Analysis*,[8] different craft activities are listed for each cognitive level.

The Developmental Frame of Reference

In the developmental frame of reference, humans are assumed to progress in an orderly way through various growth stages. The changes may be gradual and a person may show behaviors from several different stages at the same time. Different theorists have described these stages with varying emphasis and time parameters.[4,9] Illness or dysfunction is shown by the absence of age-appropriate behaviors. In other words, the sick patient fails to pass through the expected stages of development or regresses from a higher to a lower stage. Dysfunction may be caused by neurological impairment, trauma or environmental deficits. The cause is not as important as the effect on developmental function. Dysfunction is defined as the failure to master or accomplish the life tasks expected of that particular stage of development.

Activities such as crafts are thought of primarily as vehicles for attaining stage-specific behavior, for achieving mastery of a developmental stage. The treatment environment is arranged to maximize and promote development. For example, for a dysfunctional five-year-old, appropriate life tasks might include learning to get along in groups, copy letters, color within lines, use scissors and construct with materials.

An appropriate developmental environment would include materials such as wood, hammer and nails, clay, paper for copying words from the many large printed posters on the walls, and outline drawings of familiar objects to be colored, cut out and pasted. Such activities would be carried out in dyads or small groups to accomplish the task of age-appropriate socialization.[3,4,10-12]

The Role Acquisition Frame of Reference

In this frame of reference, human life is understood as a series of social roles, some held or experienced concurrently. Humans learn their roles from other people and their role behavior is influenced by their environment. Each individual is expected to learn the roles specified by the culture in which he or she lives.

Illness or dysfunction occurs when role patterns are disrupted. When traumatic or environmental factors keep people from performing an expected role such as parent, worker or friend, they are considered to be dysfunctional. When the role of patient or sick person is learned and practiced, the goal of therapy becomes assisting the individual to relearn a more functional role or in the case of chronic or terminal illness, to adapt the role so that function is maintained.

Work, activities and crafts used in this frame of reference relate to the concept of learning by doing. The tangible and immediate aspects of crafts are used by the therapist as a teaching-learning situation. Crafts can be used in environments that are simulated or natural. A simulated activity might be one in which a patient who states that he or she has no friends is asked to decide upon a handmade gift he or she might like to receive from a friend, then look at craft samples to find a similar object to make to give to himself or herself. A natural activity might be to decide on a gift to give to a prospective or real friend. In each case, the patient is learning behaviors related to the role of friendship.[2]

The Biomechanical Frame of Reference

In this frame of reference, human beings are understood to experience a specific difficulty in the form or function of body parts, which makes them incompetent to perform specific tasks. The treatment process applies simple problem solving, in that it observes how the problem affects function, measures the extent of the dysfunction, makes reasonable goals for treatment, devises methods of achieving the goals and evaluates to see if treatment methods achieve improvement.

Because the body is viewed somewhat as a machine, disease is viewed as mechanical dysfunction. Dysfunction results when endurance, strength or range of motion is not sufficient to perform a desired task. Even psychosocial or cognitive problems may be treated through the simple cause-and-effect approach. In treating psychosocial problems resulting from physical deficits, both psychodynamic and developmental principles are incorporated in treatment.

An activity such as leatherwork might be used in this frame of reference to achieve a goal gradually through the application of graded resistance. Exercises are frequently preferred to craft media in this frame of reference because they are felt to be easier to measure or control. When crafts are used, they are often seen as a way for the patient to begin to deal with his or her own mental health problems.[13]

Life-Style Performance Frame of Reference

This frame of reference is based on the concept of needs satisfaction. Humans want to satisfy their needs, to perform their own self-care, contribute to the welfare of others and be in relationships that sustain them. Thus culture, a group's design for acceptable beliefs and behavior, is an important feature of this frame of reference. Achievement of the above skills depends on cultural norms and values; consequently, culture can affect health. This frame of reference parallels the psychodynamic theories of human behavior more closely than most other occupational therapy frames of reference.

In this frame of reference, illness is defined by the inability to meet one's own needs as well as perform those behaviors expected by culture. Feelings of helplessness and being out of control, caused either by internal or external circumstances, can result in dysfunction. The origin of illness can be biomechanical, biochemical or environmental but the effect is a decrease in independent need satisfaction. This performance-based frame of reference draws on theories from sociology, anthropology, psychology, psychiatry, biomedics and biomechanics and attempts to unify psychodynamic and developmental perspectives into a single perspective. This is why many therapists find that this frame of reference is more inclusive and more adaptable to eclecticism.

The view of crafts in this frame of reference relates strongly to purpose. Exercise is seen as having a single purpose, that of body motion, while activities other than exercise may combine multiple purposes or meanings. *Doing* becomes a critical skill and *doing* in a group is the most valuable. Through doing, patients learn culturally acceptable ways of communication as well as actual task skills.[2,4,5]

A psychological theory of human behavior that fits in some ways with the life-style performance frame of reference is that of Abraham Maslow, a psychologist who focused on what people can do rather than what they cannot do. He saw human life as a hierarchical approach to satisfying human needs. Many occupational therapists use his theories, which is basically a psychological approach but is easily adapted for occupational therapy. A more thorough explanation of this theory is found in the Introduction to Chapter 7. It includes a diagram of how crafts can be conceptualized for a hierarchical satisfaction of needs.

Rehabilitation Frame of Reference

This frame of reference considers the potential for improvement in human function. Humans have many more capabilities and resources than they ever use.[14] Humans are thought to have segments in their lives such as physical, mental, social and vocational.[15,16] Each of these aspects of the human is assessed and treated independently by individual professionals. The professionals then meet as a team to share their findings and to develop a comprehensive treatment plan. This approach was the forerunner to holistic patient care.[15]

The rehabilitation approach has been traditionally reserved for the chronically ill and disabled. Their illness or dysfunction usually results from external trauma or through endogenous illness. Problems amenable to the rehabilitation frame of reference are often problems for which there is no permanent solution or cure. Activities are chosen in this frame of reference because they can challenge the patient to go beyond what he or she could do or to help him or her to reach the limit of his or her capabilities. Crafts may be used to achieve goals in physical, mental, social and vocational spheres, but work-simulated or other vocationally related tasks predominate. The patient may engage in activities of daily living (ADLs) as an adjunct to vocational roles. The current ADL approach used in many occupational therapy rehabilitation treatment settings has reduced the use of crafts as a treatment medium. Cooking is the main craft used now.[3,14-16]

Human Occupation Frame of Reference

The human occupation frame of reference takes an environmentally interactive approach. Humans are intrinsically motivated to become involved with their environments. Environmental interaction in its broadest sense is the essence of human occupation; human occupation is occupational therapy's ultimate domain of concern. Occupation is expressed as an innate need to contribute to society and participate in the culture.[9] The human being is thought of as an open system that is affected by the environment around it and in turn acts on the surroundings.

Dysfunction is defined as the lack of meaning or purpose and a failure to explore and become involved with the environment. Illness or dysfunction is not a static condition but has different levels and changes with the environment.

Activities such as crafts used in this frame of reference provide a treatment environment. The patient chooses to explore and work with materials. The treatment setting provides a variety of craft samples and materials so that the patient will be motivated to explore and achieve some mastery of the craft. Competence in a craft will result from development of skill in handling materials. Concurrently, the patient learns the role of a worker or crafts person, thus experiencing a feeling of mastery of the clinical environment. It is this feeling of competence or mastery that can be transferred to the exploration of the environment outside the hospital.[2]

References

1. Llorens, L.A. (1984). Theoretical conceptualizations of occupational therapy. *Occupational Therapy in Mental Health 1960-1982*, 1-14.
2. Robertson, S.C. (1988). *Focus: Skills for Assessment and Treatment*. Rockville, MD: American Occupational Therapy Association.
3. Hopkins, H.L. & Smith, H.D. (1988). *Willard and Spackman's Occupational Therapy*, 7th ed. Philadelphia: Lippincott.
4. Bruce, M.A. & Borg, B. (1987). *Frame of Reference in Psychosocial Occupational Therapy*. Thorofare, NJ: Slack.
5. Miller, B.R.J., et al. (1988). *Six Perspectives on Theory for the Practice of Occupational Therapy*. Gaithersburg, MD: Aspen Publishers.
6. Mosey, A.C. (1970). *Three Frames of Reference for Mental Health*. Thorofare, NJ: Charles B. Slack.
7. Allen, C.K. (1985). *Occupational Therapy for Psychiatric Diseases: Measurement and Management of Cognitive Disabilities*. Boston: Little Brown and Company.
8. Earhart, C.A. & Allen, C.K. (1988). *Cognitive Disabilities: Expanded Activities Analysis*. Pasadena, CA: Catherine A. Earhart.
9. Early, M.B. (1987). *Mental Health Concepts and Techniques for the Occupational Therapy Assistant*. New York: Raven Press.
10. Duncome, L.W., Howe, M.C., & Schwartzberg, S.L. (1988). *Case Simulations in Psychosocial Occupational Therapy*. Philadelphia: F.A. Davis.
11. Reed, K.L. (1984). *Models of Practice in Occupational Therapy*. Baltimore: Williams & Wilkins.
12. Reed, K.L. & Sanderson, S.R. (1983). *Concepts of Occupational Therapy*, 2nd ed. Baltimore: Williams & Wilkins.
13. Trombly, C.A. (1983). *Occupational Therapy for Physical Dysfunction*, 2nd ed. Baltimore: Waverly Press.
14. Kessler, H.H. (1947). *Rehabilitation of the Physically Handicapped*. New York: Columbia University Press.
15. Krusen, F.H., Koftke, F.J., & Ellwood, P.M. (1968). *Handbook of Physical Medicine and Rehabilitation*. Philadelphia: Saunders.
16. Rusk, H.A. (1971). *Rehabilitation Medicine*, 3rd ed. St. Louis: Mosby.

3

Choosing an Activity and Assessing Therapeutic Application

▼

The occupational therapy process, like the process in many other health care fields such as nursing and physical therapy, has several steps: screening and evaluation, treatment planning, implementation of treatment and reevaluation. Some say discharge planning is a last step, however, this step can logically be included in the overall treatment plan. Choosing an activity for a patient initially occurs during the treatment planning stage.

Treatment planning logically follows evaluation since a therapist cannot make decisions about appropriate treatment until the patient's functional level has been determined. A common approach to treatment planning is to list the patient's problems, prioritize the problems and compose long-term goals for the most important and/or treatable problems. Long-term goals are often thought of as the outcome the therapist would expect to see in three months to one year. For each long-term goal, the therapist then decides on a short-term objective that the patient could reasonably achieve in one week. The last step in treatment planning is usually to list activities that could help the patient accomplish the short-term objectives and consequently take steps in the direction of achieving long-term goals. Sometimes there is an additional step included in treatment plans called *rationale*. The rationale is the reasoning behind the choice of particular activities.

Another name for the rationale is *clinical reasoning*. The following list of 21 questions is intended to be used as a guideline to assist the therapist in clinical reasoning, ie, in developing a rationale for using a particular activity for a particular patient.

Questions for Guiding Clinical Reasoning

1. Which of the patient's goals/objectives can be achieved by doing this activity?
2. What patients have you had in the past with similar problems? What activities did you use with them?
3. What activity would the patient like to do? Are the patient's reasons for choosing that activity logical and reasonable to you?
4. What activity can you reasonably expect the patient to accomplish in the time you expect to work with him or her?
5. Could this activity help change the patient's habits?
6. What activity can help the patient learn new skills?
7. What activity could have an effect on the patient's underlying disease process?
8. What activity would allow the patient to use his or her remaining capabilities?
9. What activity would make use of the patient's remaining strengths?
10. Will the patient's disability require that the therapist do part of the activity for him or her?
11. What activities fit the patient's cultural identity?
12. What activities fit the patient's age and sexual identities?
13. What factors in this activity could make the patient worse rather than better?
14. Can the activity be completed before the patient is discharged?
15. Is the patient physically, emotionally and cognitively able to complete the activity?
16. Do you have the materials to do the activity or can they reasonably be obtained?
17. How easy would it be to make this activity more challenging or less demanding for the patient?
18. If you were called away before the patient completed the activity, could another therapist easily take over?
19. Is this activity appropriate for the frame of reference you are using?
20. How can you measure the patient's progress toward the goal for which the activity was chosen?
21. How will you know that the goal for which this activity was chosen has been achieved?

In summary, this list of questions attempts to guide the student or beginning therapist through the thought process that seasoned therapists often can do instantly and without apparent effort. That effortless quality usually follows frequent use of the clinical thinking process.

Developing a rationale for the activity chosen can give the therapist confidence that it indeed contributes to healing.[1-3]

References

1. Early, M.B. (1987). *Mental Health Concepts and Techniques for the Occupational Therapy Assistant*. New York: Raven Press.
2. Cynkin, S. & Robinson, A.M. (1990). *Occupational Therapy and Activities Health: Toward Health Through Activities*. Boston: Little, Brown.
3. Gambrill, E. (1990). *Clinical Thinking in Clinical Practice*. San Francisco: Jossey-Bass Publishers.

4
Analyzing and Grading Activities

▼

Activity Analysis

Occupational therapy is a doing profession. Clients and patients are involved in doing activities. There is an expectation of participation that can be either passive or active. Patients are seldom done unto as are many patients treated by other professions. Treatment in occupational therapy involves doing something. Consequently, there is a need to be skilled in analysis of what a person must do in each activity used with patients.

Over the years, occupational therapists have developed their own vocabulary to describe what they do. This has been and continues to be codified into a language we now call uniform terminology.[1] One such term that has evolved is *activity analysis*. In the 1940s, when there was a great deal of emphasis on physical dysfunction following World War Two, this term developed as a descriptive phrase for what a therapist must go through to understand what motions normally occur in different craft activities. The phrase activity analysis began to be used in texts written by American occupational therapists[2] but not by British occupational therapists.[3,4] While the concept of considering all aspects of an activity—psychological, physical, social and economic—was gradually gaining acceptance, the phrase activity analysis was not used consistently until the 1960s.[5-10] During the decade of the 1980s, Barris, Cordero and Christiaansen emphasized[11] that it is assumed "that it is more important to know how to analyze and modify activities than it is to know how to do these activities oneself." Realistically, one cannot analyze an activity one does not know how to do.

Many different methods of activity analyses have been developed since 1960. As practice issues have evolved over the decades, as the emphasis changed from physical to emotional and back to physical, as specialties in practice emerged, different analyses developed for each specialty. Even within the specializations in occupational therapy, each activity analysis has a slightly different organizational emphasis and asks for slightly different information. The trend toward holism, however, was reflected in 1988 with the development of one integrated activity analysis form.[12]

The sample blank activity analysis form presented here was developed for crafts and activities presented in this book. While the form is intended to be holistic in its approach to the activity analysis of performance components, sensory motor and perceptual skills, neuromuscular capabilities, cognition, psychosocial skills and work-related skills, it is possible to use the form to focus on only one performance area if that is all that the patient needs. To use the form in this fashion, the therapist would complete Parts I through XI and then complete the appropriate performance component section or sections. The therapist is encouraged to fill in all the information called for after each phrase. If the information asked for is not applicable to the activity, the therapist should write N/A in that space. A completed version of this sample activity analysis form is located in Appendix III.

Basic Form
    I.   Name of activity
   II.   Patient information (for a hypothetical patient)
       A. Diagnosis
       B. Age
       C. Sex
       D. Cultural identification
       E. Occupation
       F. Educational level
       G. Family situation
  III. Treatment goal for which activity is intended
  IV. Treatment setting requirements
       A. Size of room
       B. Working space per person
       C. Furniture arrangement (use diagram if necessary)
       D. Lighting requirements
       E. Equipment and appliances
       F. Ventilation and temperature

V.   Materials and tools needed; amount and cost of each
VI.   Presession preparation
    A.   By whom
    B.   Steps in preparation
    C.   Time required
VII.   Placement of tools and materials (eg, in cupboard, on table)
VIII.   Steps in craft activity (number in order and describe each step including time required)
IX.   Method of instruction (eg, demonstration, verbal directions, audio or visual aid)
X.   Opportunities for grading activity
    A.   Simpler to more complex
    B.   Complex to simpler
XI.   Precautions (eg, balance/gait or suicidal risk)

Performance Components

XII.   Sensory motor aspects
    A.   Sensory awareness/processing
        1.   Does the craft stimulate the visual system? How?
        2.   Is the auditory system stimulated by this craft? How?
        3.   Does the craft process stimulate the olfactory system? How?
        4.   Does the gustatory system receive stimulation? How?
        5.   What tactile involvement is required?
        6.   Is proprioception/kinesthesia/orientation of the body in space involved in this activity? How?
        7.   Does the craft involve vestibular/equilibrium stimulation? How?
        8.   Is temperature awareness necessary in order to do this activity? When?
    B.   Sensory perceptual skills
        1.   Is stereognosis, knowing by feel, necessary during this process? When?
        2.   Is awareness of body scheme or position of the body in space essential in this activity? When?
        3.   Does the patient need to discriminate the right from the left side in this craft? When?
        4.   Is it necessary to be able to distinguish whether forms, shapes and spaces are the same? When?
        5.   Will it be necessary for the patient to distinguish a figure or object from its background?
        6.   Will the patient be required to use depth perception to do this task? Explain.
XIII.   Neuromuscular
    A.   Which joint movements are involved? (eg, flexion, extension, abduction, adduction)
    B.   Are movements passive or active?

      C.   Which of the muscle groups are involved?

      D.   How much range-of-motion is necessary? (eg, full, limited, moderate)

      E.   Is muscle tone limiting completion of task? (eg, spasticity, flaccidity)

      F.   Is coordination fine or gross?

      G.   How will the patient be positioned? (eg, seated, standing, lying down)

      H.   How much endurance and strength are required in each position?

      I.   Is an assistive device necessary?

XIV.   Cognition

      A.   Orientation (is each of the below necessary? Why?)

          1. Time

          2. Place

          3. Person

      B.   Attention span; longest time period required for concentration on one step

      C.   Memory

          1. Short-term memory requirements (10sec. to 10min.)

          2. Recent memory requirements (hours, days, months)

          3. Long-term memory requirements (years to remote past)

      D.   Comprehension level (use either age- or grade-level performance expectations.)

      E.   Judgment

          1. Need for formulating an opinion

          2. Need to make comparisons

          3. Need for socially appropriate expression of opinions or responses

          4. Need for impulse control

XV.   Psychosocial

      A.   Opportunities for testing reality of patient's own perceptions/beliefs (eg, is my behavior/perception/belief normal?)

      B.   Opportunities for affective expression

          1. Hostility/aggression (eg, motion such as hammering, tearing, piercing)

          2. Sadness (eg, slow movements)

          3. Happiness (eg, pride, hope, laughter)

          4. Loving (eg, stroking, holding)

      C.   Opportunities for creative expression

          1. Ideas

          2. Planning

          3. Inventiveness

          4. Curiosity

          5. Use of color, shape, design

      D.   Interpersonal opportunities
          1. Needing to cooperate with
             a. the therapist
             b. another patient
             c. the group
          2. Sharing tools
          3. Increasing self-esteem
          4. Developing leadership

XVI.   Opportunities for practicing work-related skills
      A.   Taking instruction
      B.   Accepting authority
      C.   Being able to adapt
      D.   Setting goals
      E.   Planning independently/cooperatively
      F.   Performing independently/cooperatively
      G.   Showing stress management/coping skills
      H.   Demonstrating body mechanics
      I.   Timing/waiting
      J.   Counting
      K.   Making decisions
      L.   Evaluating self

Grading

Crafts can offer satisfaction at almost any functional level by either increasing or decreasing their complexity or size. By approaching each craft with a view to changing its level of difficulty, a therapist can match an activity with the treatment needs of the full spectrum of patients. Grading, as used by occupational therapists, may be defined by the Webster's[13] definition of *gradual*, which comes from the same word root:

> **gradual** adj. (1) proceeding by steps or degrees (2) moving, changing, or developing by fine, slight or often imperceptible degrees.

Many patients improve, while others may deteriorate. A craft that the patient may have accomplished or been proficient in at an earlier period may still be simplified.

This is central to occupational therapy—to match or adapt the activity to the patients. By approaching each craft with the sure knowledge that it can be made simpler or more complex according to the needs of patients, the therapist can be confident that patients can be allowed to choose a craft that fits their self-concept.

The therapist can be sure that measurable performance goals can be written and achieved for almost every craft in this text. These goals can be made with patients and discussed as a way for them to evaluate their own level of capability. This offers an opportunity to discuss how the short-term objectives of a craft project can be related to long-term performance goals. The gradability of crafts can be used to demonstrate the small steps patients must take to achieve true independence.

In the chapters that follow, examples of simple and more complex approaches to the same craft are included. In choosing a level of complexity, the therapist must first become proficient at activity analysis.

References

1. Uniform Terminology Task Force. (1989). *Uniform Terminology for Occupational Therapy,* 2nd ed. Rockville, MD: American Occupational Therapy Association.
2. Willard, H.S. & Spackman, C.S. (1947). *Principles of Occupational Therapy.* Philadelphia: Lippincott.
3. Colson, J.H.C. (1944). *The Rehabilitation of the Injured: Occupational Therapy.* London: Cassell and Company.
4. Haworth, N.A. & Macdonald, E.M. (1946). *Theory of Occupational Therapy.* Baltimore: Williams & Wilkins.
5. Council on Physical Medicine of the American Medical Association. (1947). *Manual of Occupational Therapy.* Chicago, IL: American Medical Association.
6. Department of the Army. (1951). *Occupational Therapy.* Washington, DC: US Government Printing Office.
7. Fidler, G.S. & Fidler, J.W.A. (1963). *Communication Process in Psychiatry: Occupational Therapy.* New York: The MacMillan Co.
8. MacDonald, E.M. (1960). *Occupational Therapy in Rehabilitation.* London: Bailliere, Tindall and Cox.
9. Scullen, V. (1956). *Occupational Therapy Manual for Personnel in the New York State Department of Mental Hygiene.* Albany: State of New York Department of Mental Hygiene.
10. Willard, H.S. & Spackman, C.E. (1963). *Occupational Therapy,* 3rd ed. Philadelphia: Lippincott.
11. Barris, R., Cordero, J., & Christiaansen, R. (1986). Occupational therapist's use of media. *American Journal of Occupational Therapy, 40*(10), 679-684.
12. Hopkins, H.L. & Smith, H.D. (1988). *Willard and Spackman's Occupational Therapy,* 7th ed. Philadelphia: Lippincott.
13. *Webster's Seventh New Collegiate Dictionary.* (1969). Springfield, MA: G & C Merriam Company.

5

Shall I Use a Kit or Start From Scratch?

Introduction

If we consider *from scratch* to mean *beginning by using raw materials*, occupational therapists probably never did start from scratch. In woodworking, that would have meant cutting down the tree, aging the wood and sawing it to proper thicknesses for use. In leathercraft, from scratch would have meant raising and killing one's own animals before tanning the hides. For needlework, the craftsperson would first need to make her own needle from bone or a quill before harvesting flax for linen or shearing the wool from sheep.

From our earliest professional writings, it is obvious that occupational therapists used materials that had some preparation before they arrived in occupational therapy. Of course, there was the stray therapist who may have learned a skill such as finding and preparing her own ceramic clay, but the profession as a whole benefited from the specialization of skills that are part of the industrialized age. Consequently, the purist who asserts that occupational therapists should not use kits because they do not show patients how to start from basics, is making an erroneous assumption about our past practice.

Costs of Therapist's Time for Materials Preparation

The development and structuring of funding for providing occupational therapy treatment has radically changed our ideas about what we can and should do for our patients. Up until the 1970s, most occupational therapists did not worry about who was paying for treatment. They took attendance and let the financial office deal with payment for services. Little consideration was given as to whether a patient had insurance or means to pay for occupational therapy. Service was provided on the basis of what the therapist perceived the patient's need to be.

By the mid-1970s, many hospitals had discovered that some insurance companies would pay an additional fee for occupational therapy over the rate charged for other daily care and treatments. This began to change the way we perceived our patients' needs. We had to begin to document more carefully to justify to the insurance company why a patient needed an hour of occupational therapy per day. We had to ask ourselves, "If this patient doesn't have insurance to pay for services or even for the occupational therapy supplies, will I need to charge other patients with insurance more in order to be able to provide the needed service?" Or, "If I buy supplies of less cost and quality, will I make more money for my department?" Or, "Is my job performance to be measured by the improvement in my patients or by how much money I can make in this department?"

The answer to this last question continues to come as a shock to new therapists who entered the profession because they wanted to help people. In many situations now, when a therapist is preparing materials, it means that she is not earning money for the department through chargeable patient treatment. The pressure to produce revenue may cause a therapist to choose a kit rather than grading an activity up to a more complex task by using basic craft materials.

Another aspect of this issue is group versus individual treatments and the charges and costs for both. In the time before charging for treatment became such an issue, a therapist might group several patients together and work with individual patients in a less intense way but for longer periods of time. The therapist did not need to keep a time clock running in her head. As insurance companies realized that they were being charged for these new services, they began to monitor all charges more intensively. They wanted to know how the group experience was benefiting the patient. In some cases, insurance companies refused to pay for group patient treatment unless the patient had a specific goal to improve interpersonal relations.

The guidelines for diagnosis related groups (DRGs) combined with the insurance companies' goals to monitor benefits more carefully worked to create shorter patient hospital stays. Patients' long-term goals, which had been emphasized, began to take a backseat to short-term objectives for occupational therapy patients. Therapists became more concerned with writing a goal that could be achieved in a week so they could document the improvement in the patients' chart before they were discharged.

Because of the development of this kind of payment system, health care providers saw the need to become more accountable. This accountability affected not only charges to insurance companies, but compelled occupational therapists and occupational therapy departments to spend time in revenue-producing work that involved face-to-face contact with patients in an insurance-chargeable situation instead of doing materials preparation that could not be charged. All of these developments contributed to the profession's discomfort with the word *crafts*. Previously, we knew these crafts helped people improve their health and functional independence, but now we were being asked to tell how these results were achieved, without even being allowed to use the word crafts. Crafts just were not scientific enough for a health care industry relying increasingly on evaluative testing, medication and surgery.

Space is another issue that affects whether a therapist uses kits. Storage space is not income-producing space. Formerly, when hospital stays were longer and revenue production had less emphasis, it was important to have many different craft choices available so hospitalized patients wouldn't get bored with one category of craft. Hospital stays in almost all types of treatment settings have been reduced by three quarters to one half. A much simpler inventory of craft projects is possible, requiring less storage space. Kits generally take up less space than raw materials.

Use of Aides and Volunteers

Prior to the time when charging patients for services had such emphasis, registered occupational therapists often delegated materials preparation to certified occupational therapy assistants (COTA). However, COTAs' chargeable time became as important as their supervisors' time. They were revenue-producing entities. Some therapists then used aides to prepare materials because aides could not submit insurance charges. In some institutions such as the Veterans Hospitals, aides still do some of this work.

In other institutions, volunteers are sometimes used to prepare materials for patient use. Unless the volunteers have had some experience with craft materials, they require close supervision to avoid costly waste. Consequently, prepared kits are a frequently chosen alternative.

Part

II

The Major Crafts Used Clinically by Therapists

6
Woodworking

Introduction

Woodworking has been around for thousands of years. We have used it in dwellings and for furniture. Wood has provided some of our most basic human needs—heating and cooking, weapons, shelters, sports equipment, musical instruments, sculptures used in religious ceremonies and for decoration, and transportation such as bridges and railroad ties.[1,2]

Woodworking encompasses a vast number of crafts: house building, boat building, furniture making, chip carving, making wood blocks for printing, whittling, toy manufacturing, wood sculpturing and making of small wooden containers for storage.[3]

Frequency of Use

Approximately seven out of ten therapists use woodcraft at some time. Cabinet making, furniture making and other woodcrafts are commonly employed treatment methods in work-hardening units. Wooden kits are a common project in mental health treatment.

Assessments

Formal assessments that include woodcraft are *The Work Adjustment Program;*[4] *The Diagnostic Test Battery;*[5] *Build-a-Farm;*[6] *The Interest Checklist;*[7] and *The Jacobs Prevocational Skills Assessment.*[8] The Table of Evaluations and Their Craft Components (Table 6-1)

Table 6-1
Evaluations and Their Craft Components

	Woodworking	Leathercraft	Needlecraft	Mosaics	Ceramics	Paper Crafts	Cooking	Computer	Drawing and Painting
Allen Cognitive Level Test, The		X							
Azima Battery, The					X				X
B H Battery Test				X					X
Bay Area Functional Performance Evaluation, The									X
Build-a-City						X			
Build-a-Farm	X								
Carolyn Owens Activity Battery					X				
Comprehensive Assessment Process				X		X			
Comprehensive Evaluation of Basic Living Skills							X		
Diagnostic Test Battery, The	X	X			X				X
Draw-a-Person Catalog for Interpretive Analysis									X
Fidler Activity Laboratory, The						X			X
Early and Advanced Switch Games								X	
Elizur Test of Psycho-Organicity									X
GoodEnough Harris Drawing Test									X
Goodman Battery Test				X	X				X
Gremlin Hunt, The								X	
Gross Activity Battery					X				X
Homemaking Evaluation			X						
House Tree Person									X
Interest Checklist, The	X	X	X	X	X		X		X
Instrumental ADL Scale							X		
Jacobs Prevocational Skills Test	X	X					X		
Kinetic Family Drawing									X
Lafayette Clinic Battery, The						X			
Magazine Picture Collage, The						X			
Mattis Dementia Rating Scale									X
Milwaukee Evaluation of Daily Living Skills			X						
Nedra Gilette Battery				X	X				
Nelson Clark's "Clay Test"					X				
O'Kane Diagnostic Battery					X				X
Perkins Tile Task				X					
Scorable Self-Care Evaluation, The							X		
Shoemyen Diagnostic Battery				X	X				
Street Survival Skills Questionnaire, The							X		
Tiled Trivit Assessment, The				X					
Visual Organization								X	
Work-Adjustment Program, The	X								

shows what other crafts may be included in each assessment. The Work Adjustment Program has three separate tasks: sorting/packaging, assembling mimeographed sheets and manufacturing objects that are made mostly of wood, such as bookshelves or furniture. The patient is rated on a scale from one to six on such work skills and attitudes as attendance, motivation, dressing and grooming. The results are helpful in vocational rehabilitation counseling.

In the Jacobs Prevocational Skills Assessment, there is a section called *carpentry assembly*. Clients are asked to name tools. They are then requested to use the tools to put in screws and hammer a nail. their responses and actions are recorded on a checklist in relation to coordination and perceptual-motor and cognitive performance.

Woodworking is the last of five subtests in the Diagnostic Test Battery. This battery may take several weeks to complete. The wood project to be assembled is a checkerboard. It includes a base board and a number of 2in. by 2in. squares. Some of the small wood shapes are not cut precisely. Consequently, this test involves somewhat sophisticated problem solving related to measuring the squares, counting them and staining ones that the color does not match. The project assesses perceptual function, cognitive skills, planning and discrimination.

The Build-a-Farm assessment does not formally use wood as do the previous three. Wood is included among other materials such as styrofoam, clay and construction paper, which are presented to a small group of children or adolescents with the instruction to build a farm. This is a projective test in which the patient's response to the materials is expected to reflect personality traits or psychopathology. The child's interpersonal skills are assessed by this process in which group interaction is intrinsic in the activity.

The Interest Checklist simply asks the patients or clients to rate their own interest—casual, strong or none—in 80 different activities. There are several categories that might include woodcrafts: manual arts, model building, home repairs and woodworking. The patient's or client's responses on the checklist are then used as a basis for discussion of leisure use.

Working with Wood

In the past, adapted equipment such as the bicycle saw, treadle lathe and treadle sander was a regular feature of an occupational therapy clinic. These items are seldom seen now. Some clinics have woodworking shops containing large power tools like the drill press, the table saw, and the band saw. Many clinics use only hand tools or hand-held power tools. In the following project discussions, hand tools will be described rather than power tools since hand tools are available to almost everyone. They are also less dangerous when used properly. Most woodworking tools and supplies can be purchased at hardware stores and lumber yards in the community.

Often, occupational therapists are in situations where they need to adapt equipment for their patients. For this reason, it is important for the therapist to have some skill with carpentry tools. While more commercial adaptive equipment is available every year, therapists will inevitably work with patients for whom no commercial device seems right. The therapist will need to do what we do best—*adapt*—and the adaptations often require the use of woodworking tools.

Supplies for Three-Legged Stool

A very simple kit, such as a three-legged stool, in which all the parts are precut, can be completed in two sessions (Figure 6-1). A kit like this commonly contains three legs that are each 1in. in diameter by 7in. long and a circle of 3/4in. thickness of pressed wood with a hardwood veneer and sandpaper. The round holes for setting in the legs are precut.

PROCESS
1. Sand all four pieces.
2. Finish them with paint or stain.
3. When dry, glue the legs into the inset holes.

This is a simple three-step process that does not require tools except for the sandpaper and paint brushes.

Sanding has been an important tool in the occupational therapist's treatment armamentarium for many years. In the past there were many different designs for sanding blocks to which sandpaper was attached with tacks or staples. There were those with handles on top, with cut-out holes for thumb or fingers, each planned to place a patient's hand in the desired position.

Cylindrical sanding blocks had sandpaper affixed to a 12in. length of 1 1/2-or 1 1/4in. dowelling (Figure 6-2). Such a block would be used to achieve wrist extension and flexion in all finger joints. Another aid was the sanding table (Figure 6-3), which could be raised or lowered to achieve use of different upper extremity joints (Figure 6-4).

Supplies for Pilgrim Stool

A more complicated wood project would be the pilgrim stool (Figure 6-5) so called because it was designed by our pilgrim ancestors. This small stool has five pieces. Soft wood such as pine or fir is recommended rather than hardwood such as oak. The stool has the simple rabbet joint and is assembled with screws and wood glue.

PROCESS
1. Use a carpenter's square and pencil to transfer the enlarged pattern from 1in. squared grid paper to the wood.
2. Measure and cut from 3/4in. board. Most of the sawing can be done with a handsaw (Figure 6-6) and coping saw (Figure 6-7).

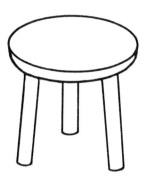

Figure 6-1
Three-Legged Stool

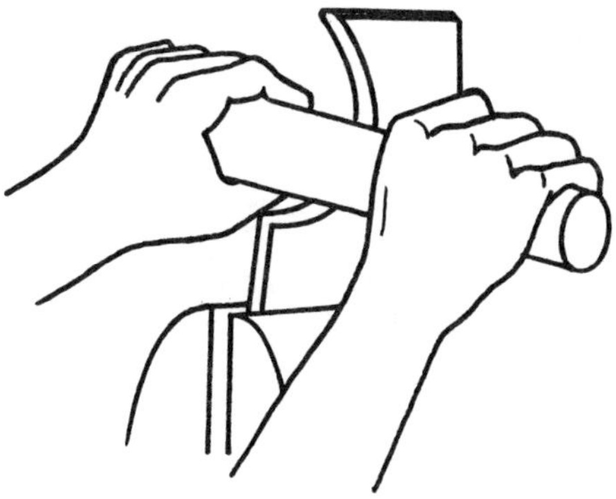

Figure 6-2
Cylindrical Sanding Block

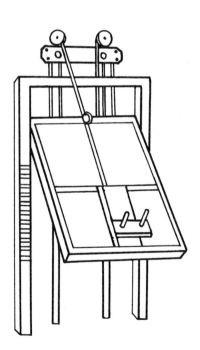

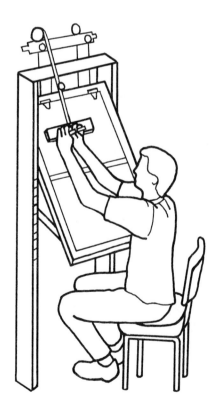

Figure 6-3
Sanding Table

Figure 6-4
Sanding Table with Patient's
Shoulder in Extension

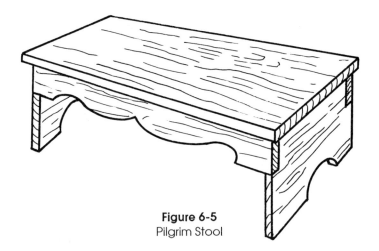

Figure 6-5
Pilgrim Stool

3. Assemble the pieces to see if they fit.
4. Sand each piece.
5. Glue the pieces together.
6. Mark and drill the holes.
7. Counter sink the screw in the rabbet joint (Figure 6-8).
8. Fill the holes with wood putty and resand or cover the holes by using wood plugs made from dowelling to resemble the wooden pegs used by our ancestors.
9. To finish, use stain, paint or one of a number of waterproof finishes.[9]

Woodcarving

Woodcarving can be quite complicated. However, an often-used craft that incorporates some similar processes is chip carving. It is a way

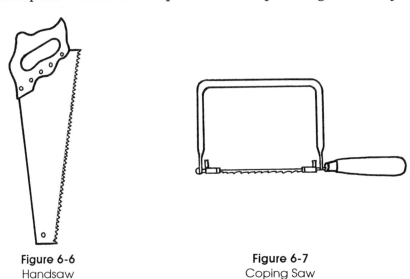

Figure 6-6
Handsaw

Figure 6-7
Coping Saw

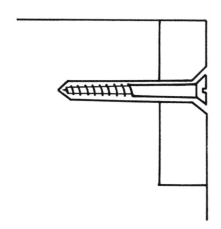

Figure 6-8
Counter Sunk Screw
in Rabbet Joint

of cutting a design into a wooden surface. The blocks used in wood-block printing are created with a similar process. In this way carving can be simplified by using scraps of boards or prepared bevelled wooden plaques. Balsawood, which is a very soft, light-weight wood works well. Pine is another soft wood that can be used.[10] Hardwood should be avoided as it is too difficult and dangerous to use in this craft. Chip carving, because of its resistive nature and because it is a constructive/destructive craft, may facilitate emotional catharsis. It requires few tools—a carving knife, a gouge, chisels and a bracer board.

PROCESS

1. Draw the design on the flat wood with a pencil.
2. Cut the outline with a carving or utility knife. (Carving tools must be kept sharp by frequent honing on an oilstone.)
3. Place a carving chisel in the cut outline, with the beveled edge facing the area to be chipped away. Press down and push away from the line (Figure 6-9). Remove the chip. A mallet may be used if the wood is very hard, but it is good to go slowly, as once the chip is out, it cannot be replaced.[2]
4. Once sufficient wood has been chipped away from the outline, use a gouge with a concave-shaped blade. Start with larger areas to be chipped away and progress to smaller, more detailed parts. Care should be taken to keep the surface a uniform depth where wood is chipped away.
5. Sand and finish the product unless it is to be used for printing. Wood is left unfinished for printing.

Main Therapeutic Applications

Physical Dysfunction

Because of the traditional identification of woodworking with masculine pursuits, this can be a valuable activity for men who have lost some of their physical capacities. While large electric power tools are not discussed in this chapter, their availability and use might assist

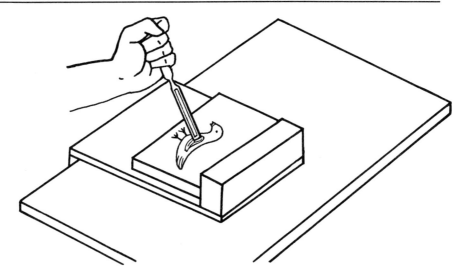

Figure 6-9
Chip Carving Against a Bracer Board

a man in compensating for lost strength. Despite the traditional association of woodworking with males, it has become more acceptable for women to do. Many women head single-parent families or live alone. They can attain a real sense of independence and achievement by learning basic woodworking. Home repairs may no longer be as intimidating for women as they once were. Home repairs, including woodworking, can be considered part of homemaking and should be included in homemaking evaluations.

Woodworking is the ideal avocational activity for the long-term patient who may be living on a disability income after discharge. The expense of the large tools makes it an important consideration to help the physically disabled woodworker find a place to work. Community schools often have woodshops that students can use. Sometimes an able-bodied hobby woodcrafter may have spent considerable money to establish a workshop and yet not use it often. A disabled woodcrafter might find such a workshop to share by advertising in the local newspaper.

Range-of-motion in the hand, finger flexion and thumb opposition, and adduction, and gross grasp can be achieved through carpentry. Wrist flexion, extension and ulnar deviation can be attained with hammering and chip carving. Flexion and extension of the elbow can be accomplished with hand drilling, sanding, hammering and chip carving. Many shoulder movements are needed in carpentry: flexion, extension, internal rotation, external rotation and scapular retraction. If a therapist is lucky enough to have any of the bicycle or treadle tools, much can be achieved with the lower extremities. By changing the height or position of the wood and tools, a therapist can achieve almost any joint and muscle movement. Weights can be added to increase resistance.

Gravity or adaptive equipment can be used to decrease resistance. The therapist is encouraged to try each movement herself and take note of which muscles are needed.[11]

Woodworking tools can be built up with foam padding for patients with weak grip. *Note:* Patients with diminished sensation, diminished circulation or immune response need to be supervised carefully as it is easy to scrape skin or to hit a finger or thumb in woodworking.

Mental Health

Because of their permanence, wood projects give a real feeling of accomplishment, which is tied to self-esteem. Woodworking's gradability from simple to complex provides for the wide range of functional levels found in mental health patients. This includes low-functioning mentally retarded individuals and schizophrenics to the often functionally unimpaired drug addict or alcoholic. Woodworking can assess the course of deterioration or recovery in a patient's cognition by illustrating deficits in perceptual—motor functioning, motor planning, problem solving, judgment, memory, and attention span.

While woodworking is often an individual skill and activity, the use of small, simple, precut kits allows it to be used as a group activity to enhance interpersonal interaction. Patients need to share tools, glue and containers of finish.

Pediatrics

From early childhood, toddlers enjoy the hammer-and-pegs toy, which develops eye-hand coordination, muscular control and object manipulation. By age three years, many children enjoy constructing with wooden blocks. Sex role differentiation occurs around this age. The masculine identification with wood can be positive. Fathers can be encouraged to include their sons in building activities. By age four years, many children envision complicated ideas but have difficulty carrying them out. Woodworking with hammer and scrap wood stimulates this kind of creativity. Normally, by age five years, a child enjoys starting something and continuing to work on it day after day. As the child begins to count and to discriminate sizes and shapes, woodworking is a natural way to use numbers in measurement and comparison of shapes.[12] Small, odd shapes and sizes of wood can be gathered at most lumber yards or cabinetmaking shops. Such wood should be checked for splinters before using it with children. They like to glue these odd pieces for sculpture. Surfaces can be painted, collaged or decoupaged.

Tongue depressors or craft sticks make nice structures. Children like to make objects that are useful. Children also like to make imaginative and symbolic objects. Some craft books include structures that may have little value or lasting interest for the child. These need to be avoided.

Woodworking from plans and drawings is too difficult for most children. They need constant one-on-one attention, which is not possible in some situations. Keep in mind, too, that in working with children, hand tools are expensive and may be underutilized in relation to their cost.

Teenagers are more likely to be able to draw and follow plans. Carved wooden sculptures will often appeal to adolescents.[13]

Geriatrics

Some of the problems common to geriatric patients are diminished memory, vision and hearing and increased pain. These factors affect their ability to do woodworking. Therapists can make adaptations for these problems. Precut kits often have only a few steps. The patient can spend some time on one step that is repetitious such as sanding or rubbing with stain. Each step is taught separately so the patient doesn't have to remember what comes next. When finishing an object, dark paint or stain makes it possible for the visually impaired to avoid missing any spots. There are some special precautions needed for the elderly doing woodcraft. The hearing-impaired patient may be unaware of how much noise he or she makes while hammering. Also, pain may keep a patient from participating.

It is easy to injure oneself with some woodworking tools. The elderly need to have particular care taken that they do not injure themselves, as they heal more slowly than younger people.

Patients in acute care, because of the crisis situation, are often not very creative. With nursing home patients, the situation lends itself more to starting with very structured activities such as the three-step kit described previously and going on to more creative projects. An elderly patient who has had some furniture-building experience may enjoy miniature reproduction. Simple craft materials such as balsawood, a single-edged razor blade and water-soluble glue can be obtained in most craft stores. Regular furniture design can be scaled down so that a weakened person can still produce fine miniature furniture.[14]

Elderly male patients often get very involved in woodcraft such as woodburning. Two or three elderly men doing woodburning together seem to stimulate each other to better performance. Woodburning requires minimal complex cognition but allows for much innovation. The patients may choose or draw their own designs. Older women are willing to do traditionally masculine projects like woodwork while men are seldom willing to do feminine crafts such as needlework.

Case Study

Paul, a white 30-year-old sign painter became unconscious after touching a boom that was in contact with live electric wires. He was working on a scaffolding 20ft. in the air. When he became unconscious, he fell 10ft. into a tree, which broke his fall to the ground. He remained unconscious for several minutes. When he regained consciousness, some men working nearby took him to the hospital emergency department. During the week he was in the hospital, he felt groggy and in pain. The physicians were unable to find any physiological reason for his pain so they referred him to a psychiatrist.

After discharge he returned to work and continued to see the psychiatrist for two years. His relationships both at work and at home deteriorated during this time. He felt he had a good job but was afraid of losing it if he took time off for treatment of his pain. He took many medications attempting to rid himself of the back pain. His temper became a problem and he often got into arguments and fights with his coworkers.

At home, his conflicts with his wife were about their children and her wish to return to work. They had two girls, ages five and three. The three-year-old had a diagnosis of cerebral palsy and was severely mentally retarded. She required almost total care. Now that the five-year-old was in kindergarten, Paul's wife wanted to return to her job as a licensed practical nurse. She had been unable to find appropriate child care for the child with cerebral palsy. The family physician and Paul's psychiatrist favored institutionalizing the three-year-old but their families were opposed to the idea. Paul was suspicious of his wife wanting to return to work. He felt her desire to work was just a cover for an affair with another man. These conflicts contributed to Paul's feelings of anxiety.

A nurse in his physician's office suggested further evaluation and referred him to the outpatient unit of a rehabilitation hospital. He was evaluated by a team including an occupational therapist, physical therapist, psychologist and vocational evaluator. The occupational therapist gave him an interest inventory and the Minnesota Rate of Manipulation test. He checked woodworking along with photography and painting on the interest inventory as activities he enjoyed. During the Minnesota Rate of Manipulation test, he was not able to tolerate sitting through all three trials. He completed only two before his sitting tolerance and concentration gave out. Despite this, he scored high on fine and gross motor coordination. In physical therapy, he was found to be unable to walk more than 1/8 of a mile. During the team meeting following the evaluations, they discussed his obvious depression.

Occupational therapy goals for Paul were to:
- Involve him in worklike activities to evaluate his future work potential;
- Increase his sitting and standing tolerance and strength; and
- Explore his avocational interests while increasing his activity level.

The therapist had Paul begin by using hand tools to make a pilgrim stool in the work-hardening program. He started very slowly, taking twice as long to do each step as it normally took.

The Saturday after he had been in the program eight weeks, he attended a craft fair with his wife. The many different kinds of woodcrafted objects he saw stimulated him to be more creative with his woodworking in the work-hardening program. The next week, he designed and made a shelf. Several other patients liked his design so well that they asked to use it to make shelves of their own. His self-confidence and self-esteem began to increase.

He attempted even more difficult projects: a bird house, toy box for his children, dog house and an entertainment center. As he became more involved, he did not want to attend physical therapy. The treadmill and the stationary bicycle just didn't motivate him like woodworking did. It was decided in a team meeting with his physician that it was time to discharge him from the rehabilitation program.

He and his wife did continue weekly visits to the psychologist for several months. Returning to his job, he found that he was able to work without pain medication. He began to use his father-in-law's garage woodshop to continue doing woodcraft.

Discussion Questions

1. How might it have been possible to discover Paul's interest in woodworking earlier in his treatment so that he might have gotten involved sooner?
2. What are some precautions you would need to observe with this patient?
3. If this patient had been a female who had the same diagnosis instead of a male would this have been an appropriate craft choice? Why or why not?
4. Make a list of your own woodworking experiences. Have you included things you may have done in elementary school, Girl or Boy Scouts, 4-H Club? How could you use some of those projects with patients?

References

1. Douglass, J.H. (1960). *Woodworking with Machines*. Bloomington, IL: McKnight & McKnight Publishing Company.
2. Scharff, R. (1952). *Handbook of Crafts*. Greenville, CT: Fawcett Publications.
3. Reader's Digest. (1979). *Crafts and Hobbies*. Pleasantville, NY: The Reader's Digest Association Inc.
4. Llorens, L.A., Levy, R., & Rubin, E.Z. (1964). Work adjustment program. *American Journal of Occupational Therapy*, 18(1), 15-19.
5. Androes, L., Dreyfus, E.A., & Bloesch, M. (1965). Diagnostic test battery for occupational therapy. *American Journal of Occupational Therapy*, 19(2), 53-59.
6. Clark, E.N. (1978). Build-a-City: Presented at 1978 Occupational Therapy Conference in San Diego, California.
7. Matsutsuya, J.S. (1969). The interest checklist. *American Journal of Occupational Therapy*, 24(4).
8. Jacobs, K. (1985). *Occupational Therapy: Work-Related Programs and Assessments*. Boston: Little, Brown.

9. Feirer, J.L. (1972). *Industrial Arts Woodworking*. Peoria, IL: Chas. A. Bennett.
10. Marshall, E.M. (1975). *Occupational Therapy: Fundamentals of Work*. Thorofare, NJ: Slack.
11. Department of the Army. (1971). *Craft Techniques in Occupational Therapy*. Washington, DC: US Government Printing Office.
12. Kaluger, G. & Kaluger, M.F. (1984). *Human Development—The Span of Life*. St. Louis: Times Mirror/Mosby College Publishing.
13. Gaitskell, C.D. & Hurwitz, A. (1975). *Children and Their Art*, 3rd ed. New York: Harcourt, Brace, Jovanovitch.
14. Better Homes and Gardens. (1966). *Stitchery and Crafts*. New York: Meredith Press.

7
Leatherwork

Introduction

It would be difficult to find a person who is not using or wearing leather or a simulation of leather: shoe, belts, hat, buttons, garments, wallets, checkcovers, notebook covers, holsters, kneepads, steering wheel covers, animal leashes, harnesses, thimbles and balls, to name just a few. Leather is our most ancient fabric.[1] From archaeology, we know that prehistoric humans used leather.[2] Uses of leather have been documented in a number of different cultures: Chinese, ancient Hebrew, Roman, North American Indian, Eskimo and early European.[1,2] We do not know as much about leather as we know about ceramics because leather has been less durable over the centuries.

An important visual construct that many occupational therapists use to attempt to understand human behavior is Maslow's Hierarchy of Human Needs (Figure 7-1). It presents the idea that our basic needs control our behaviors. If our needs are physiological, they are at the survival level; if these needs are unmet, we are then unable to attend to needs higher up on the hierarchy. Using Maslow's hierarchy, we can think in a hierarchical way about how leather was used as needs were met.

Frequency of Use

In the craft surveys, leatherwork is frequently used. Many therapists use leatherwork with their patients once per week or more; some use it daily. In the past, leather was often used to make adaptive devices such as slings and splints for patients. Commerical products have made

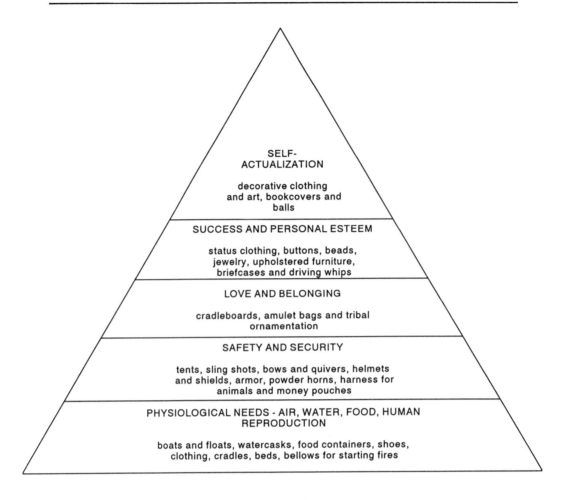

Figure 7-1
Maslow's Hierarchy of Human Needs

this unnecessary for the most part. However, a therapist's familiarity with leathercraft provides the knowledge to change or adapt commercial products when necessary.

Assessments

Leatherwork is part of the following formal occupational therapy assessments:
- The Allen Cognitive Level Test, which uses a leather lacing task to determine into which of six cognitive levels a patient fits.
- The Diagnostic Test Battery, in which a patient chooses a background pattern to engrave or tool on leather. Findings from this part of the assessment have to do with tactile perception, coordination, making and following plans, self-perception and affect.[3]

- The Jacobson Prevocational Skills Assessment has a section called *leather assembly*. The client is asked to assemble a simple leather key ring following a demonstration by the therapist.[4]

Additionally, leatherwork is included in checklist evaluationssuch as the Neuropsychiatric Institute (NPI) Interest Checklist.[5] The Table of Evaluations and Their Craft Components (Figure 6-1) shows what other crafts may be included in each assessment.

Choosing Leather

Leather comes from fur- and wool-bearing mammals; from scaly creatures like snakes, alligators and lizards; and from birds such as the ostrich. Most occupational therapists use cowhide as it is versatile and less expensive than other leathers. The unit by which it is sold is the square foot. The thickness of the leather is expressed by weight in ounces, for example: 2–3oz. weight leather is approximately 1/16in. thick, 7–8oz. leather is approximately 1/8in. thick. The weights are usually given in a range of two numbers because leather is variable in thickness even on the same piece. Many occupational therapists stock two weights, 4–5oz. for wallets and small projects and 8–9oz. for belts, purses and holsters. For the modern clinic, these two choices plus the variety of precut, prepunched kits provide the optimal selection.

Kits offer an option that is hard to ignore. They certainly save the therapist's time and consequently money and sometimes sanity in a busy clinic. If a therapist decides to buy and prepare all her own projects or to assist patients to do so, she may stock the weights of leather described above as well as lining leather, which is a different weight and texture and a larger range of laces, snaps and fasteners. A clinic treating different levels of patients will stock both uncut cowhide for the higher-functioning patient who can benefit from the challenge of starting from scratch as well as for the more disabled patient who can successfully complete a precut, prepunched kit that can sometimes have a pre-embossed design. Availability of project kits as well as skins of tooling leather, allows the therapist to grade projects appropriately for patients' functional level.

Tools

There is such a variety of leather tools available, that it is difficult to decide which ones to acquire. Nice leatherwork can be achieved with a minimum of tools:
- A rotary punch with replaceable cutting tubes (Figure 7-2);
- A 1 3/4in. by 3 1/4in. rawhide mallet;
- A 3/4in. oblong slotting punch;
- A strap cutter (Figure 7-3);

- A snap setter;
- An awl (Figure 7-4);
- Leather shears;
- A utility knife;
- A skife (Figure 7-5);
- A ruler;
- A thonging chisel (Figure 7-6);
- Round drive punches;
- An edge creaser;
- A swivel knife (Figure 7-7);
- A sponge and water dish;
- A tracing modeler; and
- Lacing needles.

The six basic leathercraft stamps are:
1. The veiner (Figure 7-8);
2. The seeder (Figure 7-9);
3. The camouflage (Figure 7-10);
4. The beveler (Figure 7-11);
5. The pear shader (Figure 7-12); and
6. The background tool (Figure 7-13).

The last three items come in a variety of textures such as smooth, lined or criss-crossed. These six stamping tools can achieve many interesting or attractive effects. Other decorative techniques involve use of plastic design templates that offer an inexpensive source for attractive designs that are quick, easy and reusable. Alphabet stamps are good for personalizing designs to emphasize a patient's identity. From this basic collection, a therapist can gradually expand the choices as new tools and materials become available. A certain symbol, such as the peace sign in the 1960s or the unicorn in the 1980s, may become a fad.

PROCESS
1. Select the design. If it is copied from a book rather than from a template, trace it with a pencil.
2. Cut the leather to the proper size.
3. Moisten the leather on the flesh (rough) side first and then on the grain (smooth) side with a damp, not wet, sponge. The grain side of the leather is observed until it returns to its original color. This will take a minute or less.
4. Place the traced design on the leather, pencil side up so that the pencil lead does not stain the leather.
5. With the pointed end of the tracing modeler, lightly press the design into the leather.

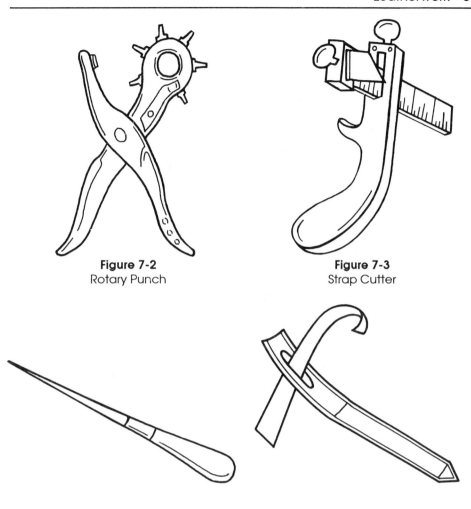

Figure 7-2
Rotary Punch

Figure 7-3
Strap Cutter

Figure 7-4
Leather Awl

Figure 7-5
Skife

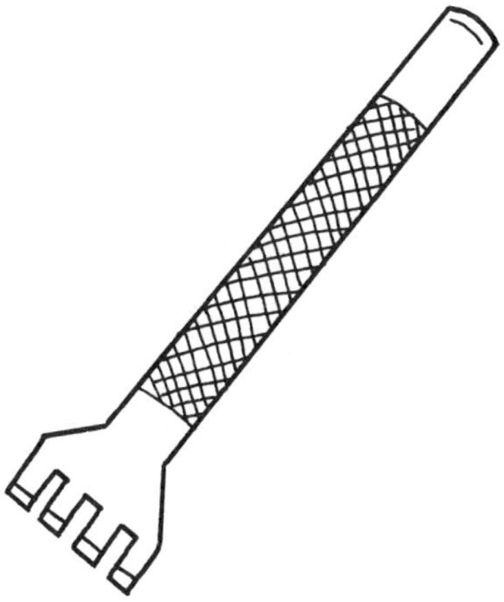

Figure 7-6
Thonging Chisel

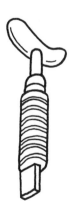

Figure 7-7
Swivel Knife

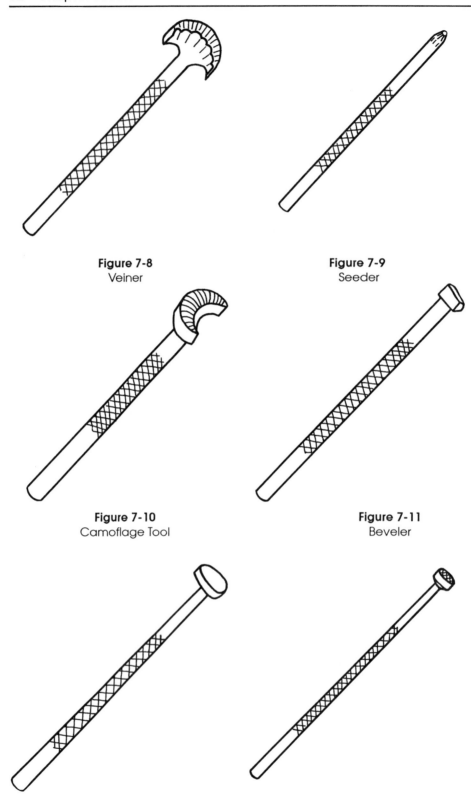

Figure 7-8
Veiner

Figure 7-9
Seeder

Figure 7-10
Camoflage Tool

Figure 7-11
Beveler

Figure 7-12
Pear Shader

Figure 7-13
Background Tool

6. Allow the leather to dry somewhat as wet leather tends to catch on the swivel knife and cause small tears and unevenness in the line. The leather should be just slightly damp when using the swivel knife for the knife to glide more easily.
7. Using a swivel knife requires practice. While the leather is drying, the patient has the opportunity to practice leather carving on scrap leather with the swivel knife.
8. After all lines are carved, the leather is again moistened with a damp sponge in preparation for tooling the design.
9. Stamping tools are held upright and struck on the flat top with a rawhide mallet. The beveler (Figure 7-11) is usually used first. The pointed end or the toe of the beveling surface is placed in the cut made by the swivel knife facing toward the center of the design. Wrist and arm movements are used rather than fingers, to manipulate the mallet in tapping the beveler as it moves along the carved line.
10. Use of the camouflage tool's half-moon shape (Figure 7-10) is usually the next step in a tooled design.
11. Next, use the pear shader (Figure 7-12), which makes contours and shading.
12. The veiner is commonly used in nature designs as its name comes from its similarity to leaf veins (Figure 7-8).
13. The seeder is a small round design (Figure 7-9) for putting centers in flowers or similar motifs.
14. Use the background tool (Figure 7-13) to impress the area around the design thus causing it to stand out more dramatically. Each of these tools is held upright and tapped with the rawhide mallet. Patients may be tempted to use a steel headed hammer. This should be avoided as a steel-headed hammer damages the chrome finish on the leatherworking tools. The steel-headed hammer can also cause the tool to puncture the leather.

These same stamping tools can be used by the patients to invent their own designs. They should practice this on a piece of scrap leather before attempting their own design on their project. A wide variety of stamping tools are available. Some are just shapes. Many are realistic pictures of objects and animals. They usually do not require the skill and concentration of leather tooling. This allows a lower functioning patient an opportunity to successfully choose and create pleasing designs.

Coloring Leather

The natural color of leather is one of its attractions. Nonetheless, patients frequently desire to add color to their designs. There are a number of coloring agents, dyes and acrylic paints. Patients should be encouraged to practice on scrap leather before attempting it on their project. Each coloring agent has its own way of covering an area. It is important for the therapist and the patient to read the label. Color can be applied by a brush, a felt or wool dauber or a fine-grained sponge. Moisture-resistant finishes are numerous: lacquers, waxes and vegetable stains with an antique appearance. Oil treatment with neat's-foot or mink oil will waterproof leather, darkening it slightly. All finishes should be applied before pieces are assembled or laced.

Lacing

Lacing is a particularly important part of leatherwork for occupational therapists because its performance may indicate strength, motor planning, visual-perceptual ability, sequencing ability and tactile perception as well as frustration tolerance. As mentioned previously, the commonly used Allen Cognitive Levels Test relies heavily on the patient's lacing performance. Because of the variety of stitches—running stitch (Figure 7-14), whip stitch (Figure 7-15), single cordovan lacing (Figure 7-16) and double cordovan lacing (Fig. 7-17)—it is easy to grade stitching up to more complex or down to simple for a patient who has regressed.

PROCESS
1. Glue the pieces together with a thin layer of rubber cement applied to edges of the surfaces to be joined. Avoid getting cement any place except on those surfaces.
2. Mark the line 1/8- to 1/4in. from the edge with a ruler and the pointed end of the tracing modeler to indicate where lacing holes will be.
3. Use scrap wood under the leather and place the thonging chisel (Figure 7-6) 1/4- to 1/8in. from the corner on the line.
4. Hit the chisel on the head with the rawhide mallet until the cutting chisels go through to the wood and can be seen on the other side. Care must be taken to hit the chisel hard enough to make the lacing slots without cutting the leather in between. The chisel must be held perpendicular to the leather.
5. Continue making these slots wherever lacing will be used.
6. Two types of needles are commonly used: the two-prong needle (Figure 7-18) and the life-eye (Figure 7-19), which does not have a traditional eye. The pointed leather lace is screwed into the threaded open end of the life-eye needle. Less commonly used are regular large-eye needles with waxed linen or nylon thread. The type of stitching chosen will determine the difficulty of the next step. The lacing pony

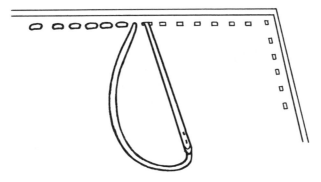

Figure 7-14
Running Stitch

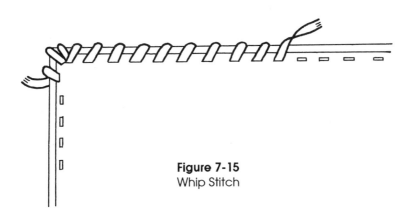

Figure 7-15
Whip Stitch

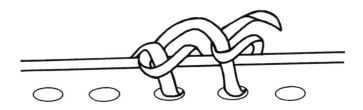

Figure 7-16
Single Cordovan Lacing

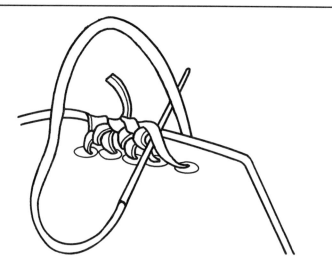

Figure 7-17
Double Cordovan Lacing

Figure 7-18
Two-Prong Needle

Figure 7-19
Life-Eye Lacing Needle

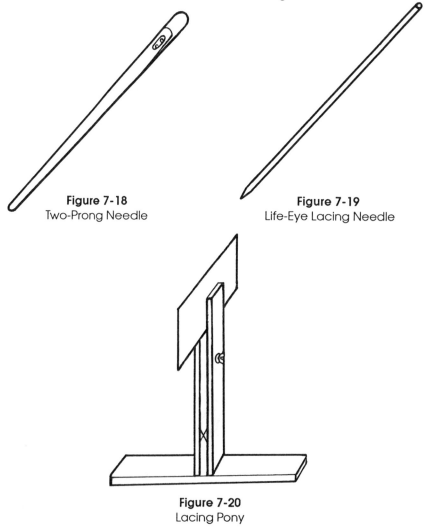

Figure 7-20
Lacing Pony

(Figure 7-20) is a tool for stabilizing a project for one-handed lacing. The pony is placed between the patient's legs with the leather held in the clamp at a comfortable working level.

The specific instructions for each individual stitch are beyond the scope of this book. They can be found in several of the texts listed as references at the end of this chapter. Link-belt kits are frequently used. Kits usually include precut pieces, a buckle and the preset snap-together buckle connector and a keeper, which is the slot through which the end of the belt slips after going though the buckle.

Main Therapeutic Applications

Physically Disabled

For the treatment of the physically disabled, leathercraft is gradable from simple to complex. It is not messy compared to wood or clay; it can be carried easily by a therapist for use with bed patients. The project will not be damaged if the patient's endurance limit is reached and the project temporarily stopped. It can be started again at almost any point. For patients in infectious disease isolation, leathercraft is an option as most leather tools can be disinfected. (Steel rotary punches may rust if not completely dried after immersion in liquid.) The leather, however, is difficult to sterilize. Chemicals in disinfectants may affect tanned leather color and suppleness. Wet leather will shrink like wet shoes dried on a heat vent. Simple projects that require few tools such as link belts or prestamped kits ready to be laced are an easy alternative for isolated patients.

For physically disabled patients who need upper extremity strengthening and endurance, leatherwork offers many opportunities. Cutting leather uses finger and thumb flexors and extensors, forearm supinators and shoulder extensors. Using the swivel knife requires static pinch, finger and thumb adduction and opposition, and wrist ulnar and radial deviation. Tooling and stamping use finger and thumb flexion, opposition and pinch, and wrist flexion and extension. Gripping a rotary punch requires finger and thumb flexion. Lacing involves the most muscle groups—finger and thumb flexion, opposition, wrist flexion and extension, pronation and supination, elbow flexion and extension, shoulder flexion and extension and abduction, and external rotation. Leatherwork can be a good method of achieving these strengthening goals while using purposeful activity to produce a pleasing product. Strengthening is achieved by gradually increasing the amount of force needed to perform the action. Slings, mobile arm supports, and the lacing pony can assist weakened joints and muscles.

The sight-impaired patient can use leathercraft as a way of

increasing tactile perception, the same tactile perception perform-ance required in using Braille reading and writing. As the patient works on the design, the impressions and contours can be felt with the fingers. These skills learned in working with leathercraft can be transferred to other activities such as dialing a telephone and identifying textures in putting clothes on right side out.

Mental Health

In the treatment of mental health patients, leather is commonly used. Easy projects such as link-belt kits or simple lacing can easily be completed by low-functioning patients. Advancement to more complex projects demonstrates in a very concrete way that a patient's function-ing is improving. Leathercraft can be used to address such common problems in mental health as concentration, attention span, memory, visual perception, fine motor coordination, self-esteem, decision making and the need to express unconscious feelings in a safe and structured activity. Natural products made of leather are valued for their scarcity as our society has come to rely increasingly on synthetics. Conse-quently, completion of a leather item can enhance self-esteem, which is a problem for almost all psychiatric patients. Traditionally, leather-work has been a male-oriented craft. It continues to be useful in that way, although many female patients enjoy it too. Benefits for the mentally retarded come in the areas of fine motor control and concentra-tion in both stamping and lacing. Lacing and stamping include both fine and gross motor control. The necessity to pay attention to where one puts the needle and where one places the leather stamp requires concentration. Increasing concentration occurs by gradually increasing the amount of time spent on the task.

Pediatrics

Leatherwork is seldom used by younger, acute care, physically disabled patients. By the time children are well enough to do leather-work, they are usually discharged from the hospital. Older children and teenagers are more likely to use leather. Kits offer satisfactory projects for pediatrics, as leathercraft is not used often enough to spend the time it takes to buy and cut the leather. Some therapists report that they seldom use leathercraft because children show little interest in it. However, it may be an appropriate assignment for angry children as they can sublimate anger through hammering. Leatherwork should be avoided for any child who is hypersensitive to sound or touch. It can be used to evaluate coordination and attention span in children and teenagers.

Geriatrics

Strength is an important consideration for leatherwork as the elderly may have diminished vigor. Because many of the tools could cause cuts and bruises, the therapist must be observant of the patients' coordination and visual perception. Cuts and bruises in some older people are difficult to heal. Many older people also have painful osteoarthritis. Gripping tools either in a pinch or grasp may aggravate the arthritis. Leather is considered by some to be a male-identified craft and nine out of ten elders are females. This is possibly why leathercraft is less often used than needlework, cooking or other "female" crafts for women patients.

Case Study

Rafael is a 23-year-old Mexican-American male who grew up in East Los Angeles. He had been brought to an alcohol and drug treatment unit run by the county. The police had picked him up outside a bar where he had been fighting. The bartender had put him out with difficulty. He and another customer had begun to argue about a debt Rafael owed. After Rafael had tried to pick up the barstool to hit the other customer, the bartender intervened and maneuvered him outside, locked the door and called the police. When they arrived, Rafael was sitting up against the wall snoring. The police had taken him to a detoxification unit. After 36 hours, they had sent him to the alcohol and drug rehabilitation unit.

During the screening interview, the occupational therapist learned about Rafael's background. His mother had been born in the United States when her mother and father were migrant workers in the fruit orchards of California. His father had come across the Mexican border illegally to find work. He was successful in that endeavor and met Rafael's mother in a Catholic Church service center. Rafael was the youngest of their eight children. He had dropped out of high school when he was in tenth grade "because it was boring." Since that time he had worked at a variety of unskilled day labor jobs. Alcohol and "machismo" had been associated in his mind as long as he could remember. While he had been arrested for drunkenness before, this was the first time he had ever had treatment. He had been engaged to marry a family friend from his neighborhood last year. The engagement had been called off after Rafael broke her jaw when he hit her during a drunken rage. Following this incident, his family asked him to leave their home as he was an embarrassment to them. They feared his unpredictable behavior.

The occupational therapist's evaluation of Rafael included the NPI Interest Checklist; the Activities Configuration; and the Allen Cognitive Levels Test. On the NPI Interest Checklist, he indicated a strong interest in leatherwork. On the Activities Configuration, he showed a very low feeling of autonomy even about the times he spent drinking.

He reported when the therapist discussed his test with him that from an early age, he had been passive in groups and allowed others to make decisions for him. He was found to be functioning at a level five on the Allen Cognitive Levels Test. His peripheral neuropathy caused some difficulty with strength and dexterity in manipulating the needle and lace. After the lacing test he told the therapist that he had always wanted to work with leather since he had seen an uncle in Mexico doing leather tooling once during a family visit.

The therapist sat down with Rafael to devise a treatment plan. Rafael told the therapist he would like to learn something that would help him get a job. After discussing the role of occupational therapy in his treatment program, they set the following short-term goals:

- To develop a daily activity plan and schedule and carry it out during the 28-day treatment program.
- To attend the daily occupational therapy goal-setting group to make and discuss achievement of daily goals.
- To increase the strength and dexterity in his upper extremities.

During the first week, Rafael was able to complete a leather belt with a western buckle for himself. He was so pleased with the outcome, that he wanted to do something more complicated. For his second project, he decided to make a shoulder bag for his mother who had come to visit him in the rehabilitation center. During this same time, he began a weight lifting program with the recreation therapist. His strength and endurance began to show real improvement. During his last week, he decided to try to make something for his father as a peace offering. His mother told him that his father was still angry with him because of his treatment of his former fiancee. After a discussion with the therapist, he decided to design and make a tool holster for his father, who worked in construction. They used the occupational therapy wrench, pliers and hammer to draw a pattern on newsprint paper. He drew his own decorative western design for the holster. It was made to fit on his father's belt as he did not know his father's waist size. On the day before he was to be discharged, it appeared as if he would not be able to finish so the therapist got the permission of the nursing staff to allow Rafael to work on the lacing that night. He came to craft group proudly displaying the finished tool holster. During the last session, they talked as a group about what they had done during these sessions. Rafael talked hopefully about a reconciliation with his father.

Discussion Questions

1. What questions might you ask Rafael at the time of his discharge to help him assess whether he had achieved his goals?
2. Can you name any other cultural group for whom leather is especially meaningful? What kinds of designs might they use?
3. If a patient chose to make a 10in. by 7in. decorative book cover, what are some assumptions we might make about him or her?
4. What leather project samples do you think might be the most important to have available in the occupational therapy clinic? What kinds of patients might be more likely to choose to make a project like the samples you named?

References

1. Reader's Digest. (1979). *Crafts and Hobbies.* Pleasantville, NY: The Reader's Digest Association Inc.
2. Stohlman, A., Patten, A.D., & Wilson, J.A. (1969). *Leatherwork Manual.* Fort Worth, TX: Tandy Leather Company.
3. Androes, L., Dreyfus, E.A., & Bloesch, M. (1965). Diagnostic test battery for occupational therapy. *American Journal of Occupational Therapy,* 19(2), 53-59.
4. Jacobs, K. (1985). *Occupational Therapy: Work-Related Programs and Assessments.* Boston: Little, Brown.
5. Matsutsuya, J.S. (1969). The interest checklist. *American Journal of Occupational Therapy,* 24(4).

8
Needlework

▬▬▬
▼

Introduction

Needlework could include everything from sewing tanned animal hides together, to sail-making for boats, to the creation of fine altar clothes for churches or intricate tapestries for castle or museum walls. In 18th and 19th century America, needlecraft was often the measure of a woman's worth. Sewing clothing for the family as well as quilting and mending were her constant occupations.[1]

Needlework, like woodcraft, includes such a vast number of activities that limits must be defined specifically for the purposes of occupational therapy. Four needlework categories are described here.

Types of Needlework

Simple Sewing

Simple sewing includes making clothing and home furnishings. Stitches in simple sewing start with the running stitch or basting stitch to the more difficult smocking, ruffling and buttonhole stitches.[2] Quilting is a particularly American craft for home decoration. Many stitches in quilting qualify as simple sewing though the designs and color combinations may be complex.[3]

Embroidery

Embroidery is a way of making a picture or design on cloth using a needle and thread. It can be either complex or simple. There are more than 80 different embroidery stitches from which one can choose in planning a design. Different yarn or floss is used; for example in crewel embroidery, loosely twisted yarn, usually wool, is stitched on heavier fabric.[2]

Knitting and Crocheting

Knitting and crocheting are both methods of using interlocking loops to make garments of clothing or articles for home use. Knitting uses two needles and is usually made in rows. Crocheting requires only one hooklike needle and stitching may be created in a round shape, square or in rows.

Needlepoint

Needlepoint is a variation of cross-stitch embroidery. It is done on a canvas back. Many of the world's fine tapestries are this kind of stitchery. Today's counted cross-stitch is a modern version of traditional needlepoint in which the design is worked by counting threads and coloring in the design with stitchery.

Frequency of Use

About one in five clinicians uses needlework weekly. Many others use needlework in treatment occasionally. It can be considered a major tool for occupational therapists, both as an activity for patients and as a method of producing adaptive equipment.

Assessments

Needlework is included in assessment of activities of daily living and self-care more often than in assessments of thinking or creativity. Three such self-care evaluations are the Milwaukee Evaluations of Daily Living Skills (MEDLS),[4] the Homemaking Evaluation in *Occupational Therapy for Physical Dysfunction,*[5] and the Activities of Daily Living Evaluation.[6] The Neuropsychiatric Institute (NPI) Interest Checklist also includes this craft.[7]

The MEDLS is an assessment of daily living skills for the chronically mentally ill. It has 20 subtest categories. In the MEDLS, under the category *maintenance of clothing*, patients are given a needle, thread, scissors and a shirt with a button missing and told to sew on the button. They are scored on whether they are able to complete all or part of the task in each subtest category.

The Homemaking Evaluation,[5] designed to be used in rehabilitation settings, includes sewing as one of seven major areas. The evaluation is a checklist to be completed by the therapist at the beginning of rehabilitation treatment and again at discharge. It is administered over several sessions.

The Activities of Daily Living Evaluation has a section on hand activities that includes basting and sewing on a button. This evaluation was adapted from one used at the Hartford Easter Seal Center.

The NPI Interest Checklist is filled out by the patient. It asks the patient to rate his or her interest as casual, strong or none, in 80 activities. Sewing, needlework, mending and knitting are on the list. Two other activities, decorating and making clothes, may include needlework. Informal needlework evaluations can identify functional levels of eye-hand coordination, fine motor coordination, sequencing and motor planning.

Supplies

One of the simplest stitches used in kits is cross-stitch. It has a long history with people who were trying to improve their eye-hand and fine motor skills. Many 18th century girlhood samplers used mostly cross-stitch.[1,8] While a high-functioning patient may be able to concentrate to count the stitches for the popular counted cross-stitch patterns, many patients will find it too difficult. The stamped cross-stitch kit or precut plastic canvas that has preprinted color codes offers a good alternative. Additional tools needed in needlework are both left- and right-handed scissors; thimbles; different sizes of embroidery hoops, including a three-way hoop that can stand on a table, be held between legs or clamped to table and used by one-handed patients (Figure 8-1); and an assortment of embroidery and crewel needles.

PROCESS

1. Place the bottom section of the hoop under the part of the stamped design where you want to start.
2. Press the top of the hoop over the cloth and the inner hoop. This stretches the fabric so it is easy to see the design.
3. Cut off a 14in. piece of cotton embroidery floss.
4. Separate the six strands in two so there are two strands with three threads in each.

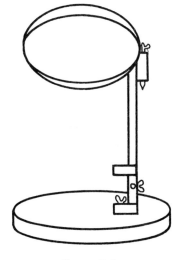

Figure 8-1
Three-Way Embroidery Hoop

5. Thread the needle. Embroidery needles have larger eyes so all strands can fit through. It may be necessary to use a needle threader, which is an important aid for most clinics (Figure 8-2). Pull the thread one third of the way through.

6. Knot the longest side on the end. Expert embroiderers do not knot their threads but for most patients it is necessary to knot the thread to keep it from pulling through.

7. From the back of the cloth, push the needle up through the end of one cross and down on the other end; then up on the other line of the same cross and down (Figure 8-3).

8. Continue this process on each cross.

9. When the thread gets short, approximately 4in., make a knot by going over and under floss strands on the back several times.

10. Cut off the excess thread leaving 1/4in. to 1/2in. after the knot.

11. Change floss colors as indicated on schematic directions included in the kit.

12. Move the hoop when the thread gets too close to the edge to work comfortably.

13. When the stitching is finished, remove the hoop.

14. Iron the picture flat. It is then ready to frame, to be sewn to a pillow cover or otherwise finished.

To add more complexity, patients can draw their own design and transfer it to embroidery cloth or canvas. Another way to vary a design is to use applique. A figure cut from one kind of fabric is sewn to another piece of cloth. A variety of stitches may be used to stitch the figure down. It can be stitched down using a buttonhole stitch on the sewing machine or by hand.[9]

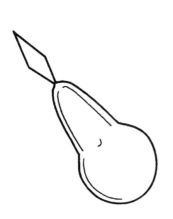

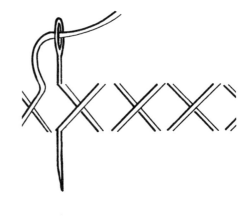

Figure 8-2
Needle Threader

Figure 8-3
Cross-stitch with an Embroidery Needle

Main Therapeutic Applications

Physical Dysfunction

Because needlework is most often identified with women, its use is slightly limited. While a few men will attempt it; only those with a strong sense of self are willing to risk doing a traditionally female craft.[10] Needlework is the kind of craft that can be done easily by bed patients. Small projects require little expenditure of energy and can be done by very weak patients. It can be stopped whenever the patient is fatigued and started when the patient is refreshed. Because the materials are inexpensive, they can be left in the room of patients in infectious isolation. Scissors can be easily sterilized with disinfectants if necessary. The therapist needs to make sure the scissors are completely dry so they do not rust.

Most of the joint and muscle movements in needlecraft are in the fingers and hands. However, needlework involves some shoulder internal and external rotation, elbow flexion and extension, forearm pronation and supination, wrist flexion and extension, and radial and ulnar deviation. Many severely disabled arthritics still enjoy needlework as it does not require strength and consequently does not hurt their joints. The patient experiences less pain when concentrating on a craft such as needlework.[11] If an arthritic patient uses a joint continuously in one position, it is possible for the stress to further damage an inflamed joint. Precautions need to be taken to avoid this. This craft is not good for the visually impaired as they cannot see patterns to stitch.

Mental Health

Embroidery can be very structured as in cross-stitch or it can be a challenging, creative experience. For depressed, low-functioning patients, needlework can be used in the acute stage of the illness as it requires little exertion. Most depressed patients complain of fatigue but needlework is seldom a fatiguing activity. Historically people have used it for relaxation such as in quilting. For hostile patients, the cutting and piercing parts of the needlework process may help them turn their hostility to constructive use. The striving for repetition and preoccupation with detail that afflicts the obsessive compulsive patient can be easily satisfied through needlecraft. Stitchery can make constructive use of these otherwise negative behaviors. The mentally retarded can enjoy and benefit from the repetitive possibilities of needlework. They can learn one step and repeat it many times.

Pediatrics

Young children ages five or six years may not have received the message that this is a female craft. It is valuable for both sexes as it involves many perceptual and fine motor skills that children need to develop such as eye-hand coordination. Sewing cards or cardboard with perforated holes along the outline of the picture are often used for beginning sewers. While it can be repetitious, it need not be. Perhaps the best way to present it to children is that stitchery is another way of drawing or picture making. They can be encouraged to draw an outline on cloth and then to stitch on that line. Burlaps or other coarse cloths are appropriate for children's stitchery. Large plastic needles are good to use on burlap. Other less coarse cloth requires metal needles that should be used cautiously as they are usually sharp. If a therapist is going to do such a project with a group of children, it may be best to cut the yarn and thread all the needles before the children arrive as they are seldom able to sit and wait for their turn for help from the therapist in threading their needle.[12] Projects appropriate for children of different ages and adolescents include wall hangings, hand puppets, placemats or simple doll clothes. Children enjoy embellishing their creations with beads, buttons, sequins or iron-on patches.

Geriatrics

Many elderly females have sewn and mended for themselves and their families throughout their lives. While women will often do a traditional male craft, few men will participate in female-identified crafts such as needlework. Because women have habitually stitched from necessity and for recreation, as in quilting, it is usually easy to get them to participate. They may also have a preferred type of needlecraft that they have done in the past. If so, this is probably the best medium for them to work in.[13] If vision is a problem as it often is for the elderly, using bright colors on white will be helpful. The contrast makes it easier for them to see. A clamp-on magnifying glass may be attached to the edge of the table if necessary. People with circulation problems common in diabetes need to be careful not to stick themselves with the needles as they may develop infections. Sometimes, demented elderly use scissors to damage something such as cutting their own clothes or bed clothes. Precautions should be taken to prevent this.

Case Study

Alice was 49 years old when she discovered a lump in her right breast. She had gotten out of the habit of breast self-examination after she went to work. Consequently, her breast cancer was quite advanced when the biopsy was done and the cancer was diagnosed. Cancer was found in her axial lymph nodes. Because Alice had not agreed to a radical mastectomy before the biopsy, she had to be rehospitalized for this major surgery. Her local surgeon referred her to a cancer specialty hospital in a nearby city. The occupational therapist there was an important member of the treatment team. She paid a visit to Alice for a screening interview the day before Alice was to undergo the radical mastectomy. This was considered an important part of the preventive medicine emphasized in the specialty hospital. The therapist hoped to prevent postsurgical complications. She learned that Alice had four daughters and had worked as a bookkeeper before she was married. After the girls were in school she did the bookkeeping for her husband's farm feed and seed store. When she was 46, her husband divorced her and married a local school teacher. Alice had been devastated by this unexpected turn of events. For a year, she kept working in the business of her ex-husband because she was afraid she was not skilled enough to do the complex computer bookkeeping required in most businesses. A friend persuaded her to take a computer class at the local junior college. Her computer teacher helped her find a job in the patient accounts department of the local hospital. Several months later she discovered the lump in her breast. Her daughters rallied to her support. Three of them lived within 50 miles. The occupational therapist queried Alice about her hobbies and learned that she had sewn many of her girls' clothes as they grew up. Recently she had been making doll clothes for her six-year-old granddaughter. They agreed that doll clothes might be a good activity for her to continue to work on during the five to ten days she was expected to be in the hospital. The occupational therapist and Alice made the following goals:

- To prevent right shoulder contracture.
- To prevent right upper extremity edema.
- To prevent depression.

The occupational therapist visited Alice soon after she returned to her room from the recovery room. The next day after checking her range of motion, she started Alice on some mild shoulder exercises and helped her cut out the pieces for a doll dress. Alice was medicated for pain. The occupational therapist instructed Alice about steps to take to prevent edema and infection in her right arm. Needle punctures need to be avoided as they could cause infection. Since her lymphatic system in that arm had been interrupted, she was much more vulnerable to wound infection, which could be quite serious for her. Alice's surgical incision was healing well. She worked much of the time on the doll wardrobe for her granddaughter. She became immediately involved in the mastectomy patients' support group, Reach for Recovery. At the time of discharge, she had increased her shoulder flexion 15 degrees since the day after surgery. From time to time, when Alice returned to the cancer specialty hospital for her chemotherapy and radiation treatments, she visited her occupational therapist. She appeared to have adapted well to her condition. Sewing had become a social enabler for her, as she was now making doll clothes to be sold in a church bazaar.

Discussion Questions

1. What craft might the occupational therapist have suggested that would have involved shoulder flexion so that Alice could have used an activity rather than an exercise to achieve this movement?
2. Which needlecraft would be the least likely to need precautions to avoid a needle puncture wound?
3. If Alice had developed a staphylococcus infection in her surgical incision and was put into isolation so other patients could not contract the infection from her as is sometimes the case, what would you do so that she could continue to participate in this activity, which was so good for her?

References

1. Banks, M. (1979). *Anonymous Was a Woman*. New York: St. Martin's Press.
2. Carroll, A. (1947). *The Good House Keeping Needlecraft Encyclopedia*. New York: Rinehart & Company.
3. Reader's Digest. (1979). *Crafts and Hobbies*. Pleasantville, NY: The Reader's Digest Association Inc.
4. Leonardelli, C.A. (1988). *The Milwaukee Evaluation of Daily Living Skills: Evaluation in Long-Term Psychiatric Care*. Thorofare, NJ: Slack.
5. Trombly, C.A. (1983). *Occupational Therapy for Physical Dysfunction*, 2nd ed. Baltimore: Waverly Press.
6. Pedretti, L.S. & Zoltan, B. (1990). *Occupational Therapy: Practice Skills for Physical Dysfunction*. St. Louis: Mosby.
7. Matsutsuya, J.S. (1969). The interest checklist. *American Journal of Occupational Therapy*, 24(4).
8. Creekmore, B.B. (1968). *Traditional American Crafts*. New York: Hearthside Press.
9. Better Homes and Gardens. (1966). *Stitchery and Crafts*. New York: Meredith Press.
10. Department of the Army. (1971). *Craft Techniques in Occupational Therapy*. Washington, DC: US Government Printing Office.
11. Council on Physical Medicine of the American Medical Association. (1947). *Manual of Occupational Therapy*. Chicago: Author.
12. Gaitskell, C.D. & Hurwitz, A. (1975). *Children and Their Art*, 3rd ed. New York: Harcourt, Brace, Jovanovitch.
13. Gould, E. & Gould, L. (1971). *Crafts for the Elderly*. Springfield, IL: Charles C. Thomas Publisher.

9
Copper Tooling and Metal Craft

Introduction

While metal and its uses were discovered by humans thousands of years after wood, ceramics and leather, it was such an important development that we have named an era after it—the Iron Age as compared with the Stone Age or Computer Age. Metal working has existed at least 12,000 years. Copper, along with gold, probably was discovered first. Copper is an element that is very malleable. It was hammered into utilitarian and decorative objects. The copper tooling we do today has a long history of use.[1] Other metals such as gold, silver, bronze, iron, pewter, and aluminum have been crafted but in modern occupational therapy clinics, copper and tin are most likely to be used. Tin is also an elemental metal. The occupational therapists' use of these two metals will be emphasized in this chapter.

Frequency of Use

In studies of crafts used by occupational therapists, there were two categories that involved metal craft: metal hammering and copper tooling.[2] Almost half of all clinics use metal craft. This makes it an important skill for new therapists to have.

Assessments

No formal assessments were found to include metal work. Because metal work is new to most patients, they would have to learn every step before it could be performed. Consequently, this probably requires more time than many therapists have for the evaluation process and could narrow the range of skills that could be evaluated. Danger may also be considered as a factor for excluding metal work in task evaluation batteries. Patients could very easily cut themselves on the sharp metal edges.

Types of Metal Crafts

Tooling is a method of making a design on a sheet of metal foil. Metal foil comes in copper, aluminum, silver and gold-colored aluminum. The thickness of the metal foil or sheet is expressed in the term *gauge*. Most tooling is done on 30- to 40-gauge metal. The thicker the foil the lower the number. Copper is most commonly used probably because of its malleability and stretchability.

Embossing is a method of working the metal from the back of the foil to raise the design on the front. Chasing is the same process done from the front of the foil. When both are combined to get a picture it is called repoussé, which means worked from both sides. All three of these methods are included in the term *copper tooling*.[1]

Metal can also be soldered, riveted, cut, bent, etched, cast or enameled. Because of the infrequency of use of most of these techniques in occupational therapy, they will not be explained further here.

Tooling

Supplies and Tools

Supplies for copper tooling include:
- 36-gauge sheet copper;
- Tracing paper and pencil;
- Plastic picture templates;
- Plasticine clay;
- Steel wool;
- Liver of sulfur;
- Water;
- Lacquer;
- Lacquer thinner;
- Masking tape; and
- Newspapers.

Tools are:
- A modeling tool (leather tracing modeler can be used);
- Sharpened hardwood dowels for tracing;

- Tongue depressor;
- Brush for liver of sulfur;
- Brush for lacquer;
- Dish for liver of sulfur;
- Dish for brush cleaning; and
- Metal shears.

The process described here will be for patients using their own designs, however the process using templates is similar but simpler.

PROCESS
1. Trace the design onto the tracing paper.
2. Cut the copper to the correct size.
3. Cover all the edges with masking tape to prevent cuts from sharp edges.
4. Tape the tracing paper to the metal.
5. Place this on a 1in. thick stack of newspapers.
6. Using the sharpened wooden dowel to trace evenly over all the lines to lightly impress the design into the metal foil.
7. Remove the tracing paper.
8. Retrace the line with the blunt point of the modeling tool.
9. Turn the copper over. Next use the spoon end of the modeling tool or a dowel with a rounded end to begin in the middle to slowly and evenly press all the parts of the design that are to be raised. Starting at the edge may cause folds in the metal. Avoid working in only one area as that copper will stretch and wrinkle. Work over the whole area.
10. Turn the copper over frequently so the raised design is facing up and flatten out the background by pressing it against the hard table top with the same tool. Alternate working on the front and the back. The important thing to remember is to work slowly and evenly over the whole area to avoid stretching one section more or making a hole in the copper.
11. When the design is raised to its completed height, fill in the reverse side of the impression with plasticine, an oil-based clay, smoothing the clay slowly and evenly to fill in the back of the raised surface.
12. Turn the copper over and with a pointed tool gently impress in the detailed lines of the design on the front.
13. Lightly go over the front of the copper with fine steel wool to clean off any dirt or oil from the tooling process. Be careful not to touch the copper after this as body oil will resist the liver of sulfur.
14. Most liver of sulfur comes in a solution form now but if it is purchased in lump form, dissolve a pea-sized lump in one quart of water.

15. Dip the copper in this solution or if the copper is too big to fit in the pan it can be applied with a brush. Liver of sulfur fumes can be annoying as it is the typical rotten eggs smell. People with allergies or respiratory problems need to be careful to avoid these fumes.
16. After the metal is dry, buff the front of the design with fine steel wool. This will allow the black oxidation from the liver of sulfur to remain in the crevices and provide contrast for the raised design.
17. After the desired polish and contrast is achieved on the front, the piece should be covered with a thin layer of lacquer that can be applied with a brush or as a spray.
18. The lacquer brush should be cleaned with lacquer thinner followed by soap and water.

Tooling done on plastic templates is the same except it leaves out the steps of tracing on paper and onto the copper because the design is already on the plastic template. Tape the copper to either the front or back of the template, whichever side has the greatest detail. Press the copper into the grooves and depressions of the template by first going over the whole surface with a blunt tool or with a tongue depressor working from the middle toward the edges. Then gradually decrease the bluntness of the tool and begin to emphasize the details. If the design seems indistinct in any sections, turn the template over to see what details need to be emphasized. For the lower-functioning patient, it may be better to tape the copper to the back of the template so the depressed design can be filled with clay before it is removed from the template. Otherwise, the process is the same.[3,4] The finished tooling may be mounted on wood using copper escutcheon pins, or it can be placed in a picture frame.

Hammering

Hammering a flat metal sheet to shape is called planishing. The process toughens the copper and gives it a texture.

Tools and Supplies
- Concave wooden mold;
- Rawhide, rubber or wooden mallet; and
- 20- to 24-gauge copper disk.

PROCESS
1. Center the copper disk on the mold.
2. With a few blows of the mallet, define the edge of the concave area under the disk (Figure 9-1).
3. Then hit with hammer, moving in a spiral outward from the center until the desired shape and texture are reached.[1,3]

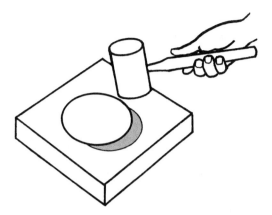

Figure 9 -1
Mallet, Copper Disk and Wooden Mold

Chasing and Piercing

Chasing means make an indention on the front of the piece without actually piercing the metal. Another kind of metal working is nail punching or piercing of the design. Both can be done on either copper or tin sheets, on tin pie plates, or tin coasters.

Tools and Supplies

Few tools are required:
- A Phillips screwdriver or nail and hammer;
- Piece of scrap wood; and
- Traced design.

PROCESS

1. Affix the traced design to the top surface of the metal.
2. Place the metal on the wood.
3. Depending on the thickness of the metal and whether chasing or piercing of the design is planned, use either a sharp nail for piercing or a blunt nail or phillips screwdriver for chasing. Position the nail or screwdriver and gently tap it.
4. Repeat until the outline of the design is complete.

Experimenting on a scrap of the metal is recommended before actually starting to work on the design. Nail punching is in an old American craft used in making the panels on pie safes and other food storage cupboards. It lets air in but keeps mice and roaches out. Nail punching kits offer opportunities to create objects that look antique.

Main Therapeutic Applications

Physical Dysfunction

Often a goal in tooling is strengthening of finger and hand flexors and the three-jaw chuck grip. Adaptations for poor grip can easily be made by using built-up tools, using a larger sharpened dowel for a modeling tool or using lighter gauge metal. Because of the concentrated static contraction of finger and hand muscles, a patient may need frequent rest periods. Nice results can be achieved even by a patient who has poor muscle strength and control in the hand. It is a quiet activity that requires little space. This craft can be performed by patients using only one hand. The therapist will need to tape down the design to be traced and over it the paper for the metal tracing. A template can also be taped in place for the one-handed patient. Liver of sulfur, steel wool and lacquer can also be applied in the same way. Patients will need to use gloves to protect their hands when using steel wool. Those for whom infection is a major threat such as diabetics, need to have special precautions taken because copper tooling has so many hazards for skin cuts or punctures on the sharp metal edges or from the steel wool. Liver of sulfur is corrosive to the airways and skin so it is best to use gloves when handling it and use a well-ventilated space. It may be necessary for the therapist to apply the liver of sulfur in a room away from patients with respiratory ailments. Copper tooling either with a template or the patient's own design can be used with blind or partially sighted patients. They can feel the contours of the picture in the same way they feel the dots for Braille reading. Again, precautions need to be taken to cover all sharp edges with masking tape, as the blind person is unable to observe the dangers visually. Bed patients can do copper tooling, but it may be advisable to use the liver of sulfur and steel wool out of the bed on a bedside table.

Hammering a metal sheet into a mold involves elbow flexion and extension and wrist ulnar and radial deviation. These motions need to be chosen with care so that a weak joint is not overtaxed or inflamed by excessive motion or impact.[3,5-8]

Mental Health

Because copper tooling on templates is a success-assured activity, many occupational therapists in psychiatric settings use it. Self-esteem is a problem for a large number of psychiatric patients. Copper tooling offers a project with a successful outcome and success is tied to self-esteem. This craft can be graded from a simple, small template to a larger, more complex template; from a simple, traced design, to a more complex design and finally to a creative design composed by the patient. Copper tooling can be used to focus on attention span, ability to stay within limits, to sequence steps, or to make decisions. If a variety of templates are available to choose from, patients who feel that many choices have been denied them in the hospital find they have a choice in a situation where they can exert some control. A patient with destructive behavior may find this rather controlled destructive/constructive craft to be a good way to sublimate harmful hostile urges. For the depressed patient, the no-fail aspect of copper tooling may be the most important. Most depressed patients have some measure of decreased self-esteem. This activity usually will not let them fail again. The slow repetitive movements are ones depressed patients are able to do despite their fatigue. The sharp edges of the copper, however, may be a temptation for self-injurious or suicidal patients. Patients who undergo electroconvulsive therapy (ECT) who may have memory problems, will have little difficulty with this simple craft.[9]

In the case of some schizophrenics, the structure offered by tooling a template is helpful. The limits are well-defined for those schizophrenics for whom boundaries are difficult to perceive. The activity does not require much concentration or thinking, processes that are difficult for some schizophrenics. The here-and-now quality of this activity in which the patient is able to immediately see results often helps schizophrenic patients exercise their own reality testing. Patients with organic mental disorders benefit from copper tooling for many of the same reasons as schizophrenics—it requires few cognitive processes and yet provides a good outcome for the patient.

Manic patients who have expansive behaviors can have inherent controls for their hyperactivity. The obvious guidelines of a template help them provide a control for themselves. The resistiveness of the copper can provide a controlled outlet for the excess energy. The patients can quickly complete the activity. This fact alone may keep them from stopping in the middle as they are easily distracted and lose interest quickly.

Traditionally, in hammering metal, the goal in mental health has been to externalize hostility and anger and thus turn both to a constructive activity. However, in some cases, these negative emotions are sometimes increased rather than decreased through a destructive/constructive craft.[3,10,11]

Pediatrics

With children, using copper tooling on templates ensures a successful outcome. However, creativity is greatly reduced. For small children, simple drawing is better as it allows for self-expression. However, older children or teens may be able to design a pattern with enough contrast to provide an interesting creative opportunity. The same precautions (eg, self-injury) that apply to adult physically and mentally disabled patients should be observed with children and adolescents. The gross motor aspect of hammering often appeals to children.

Geriatrics

Again, the no-fail feature of tooling on a plastic template makes this craft attractive for therapists working with the elderly. This activity is appropriate for the diverse nursing home population.[12] It is age appropriate, providing adult gratification with minimal cognitive requirements. With geriatric patients it is probably better to use the precut foil sheets rather than rolls of copper foil as it decreases the steps that an elderly person must remember. This also decreases the chances of inadvertent self-injury. The elderly need special precautions because they heal more slowly. Liver of sulfur may cause patients with vision problems to complain of eye irritation. Some older people may have difficulty seeing the design on the shiny metal surface.

It is often best to start patients new to crafts with this kind of simple activity, however a danger is, once elderly patients have begun to rely on a pattern, it may be difficult to break them of the copying habit.[13]

Case Study

Mabel was a 78-year-old white patient who was admitted to the geriatric unit of a psychiatric treatment program. She was brought to the unit by her son and daughter-in-law after being referred by her internist. She appeared clearly depressed but her psychiatrist in the hospital wanted to rule out possible dementia as the two illnesses so often have similar symptoms. The occupational therapist was a key member of the evaluation team because he was so often able to determine whether functional deficits were truly cognitive or emotional.

The day after her admission he performed a screening interview. Halfway through the session, her daughter-in-law joined them. She was able to add helpful information. Mabel was born and raised near the same city in which she was hospitalized. She had married her childhood sweetheart, who was a farmer, two days after she graduated from high school. Within six years, they had five children. Mabel assumed a great deal of responsibility on the farm in addition to her roles as homemaker and mother.

Involvement in the church was an important aspect of their rural community. After the children were all gone from home, she and her husband continued to farm the land. They were disappointed that one of the children had not chosen to take it over for them, but it never occurred to them to sell the farm and retire. One year ago, her husband died following several years of struggle with congestive heart disease. She had cared for him and run the farm during those years. Following his death she had gradually started to go downhill, to be less involved in the farm operation, to avoid community and church events and to be more dependent on her son and his wife. Recently she had stopped taking an interest in her self-care. Her son and his wife were the only ones of her family still living nearby. A decision was made on the telephone with her other children for her to move to the nearby city to live with her son and his wife. Her condition had worsened despite the fact that she was getting more medical attention.

The following day, the occupational therapist evaluated Mabel's sensory functions, hearing, vision, smell, taste and touch. He asked the female certified occupational therapy assistant (COTA) to evaluate her on dressing and grooming. During these evaluations, the patient had repeatedly said "I can't remember anything." She responded "I don't know" to most questions. It appeared that she just did not want to make an effort. She had some hearing loss, especially in locating the source of sounds. Her taste and smell discrimination were somewhat diminished but still functional. Her vision was adequate when she was reminded to put on her glasses. There were no tactile deficits. She dressed and groomed herself independently but needed many prompts and encouraging remarks from the COTA. The occupational therapist made the following goals for Mabel:

- To increase her self-esteem;
- To increase her activity level; and
- To develop motivation for self-care.

The occupational therapist asked the COTA to start Mabel out on some copper tooling.

Initially, Mabel tried to get the COTA to choose a template design so the COTA said Mabel could choose from among three: the praying hands, the madonna and the ballerina. She chose the praying hands. The COTA helped her tape the precut copper foil on the back of the template. Mabel started to work the impression but by that time the first session was over. The following day she completed the tooling and filled the back with plasticine clay. The following day she applied the liver of sulfur. By the time it was dry, the session was over. During third session she wore gloves while she polished off the black oxidation. Then she lacquered it and at the fourth session, she put the precut cardboard frame over it. She seemed pleased with her effort despite the statement "I would have done better two years ago." With the COTA's help she hung the copper tooling in her hospital room. Mabel asked to copper tool the ballerina to give to her granddaughter.

The physician's final primary diagnosis of Mabel was depression though he felt there was some cognitive loss as well. When she was discharged after 14 days in the hospital, Mabel told the occupational therapist and COTA that she planned to hang her praying hands in her room at her son's home where it had been decided she would live permanently. She continued in outpatient therapy with the physician. Occasionally, she stopped to visit with the COTA and told her that at the local senior citizens' center, she did another copper tooling before she decided to move on to more challenging projects in the craft room.

Discussion Questions

1. Would it have been better to encourage Mabel to try a different craft for her second project?
2. Considering Mabel's sensory deficits, can you think of a craft that might have been more appropriate?
3. If you were to use copper tooling with an HIV patient, what would the hazards be for the patient, for the therapist or for the other patients? What precautions should be taken?

References

1. Reader's Digest. (1979). *Crafts and Hobbies*. Pleasantville, NY: The Reader's Digest Association Inc.
2. Barris, R., Cordero, J., & Christiaansen, R. (1986). Occupational therapist's use of media. *American Journal of Occupational Therapy*, 40(10), 679-684.
3. Department of the Army. (1971). *Craft Techniques in Occupational Therapy*. Washington DC: US Government Printing Office.
4. Griswold, L. (1931). *Handicraft*. Colorado Springs, CO: Outwest Printing and Stationary Company.
5. Department of the Army. (1951). *Occupational Therapy*. Washington DC: US Government Printing Office.
6. Dunton, W.R. (1945). *Prescribing Occupational Therapy*, 2nd ed. Springfield, IL: Charles C. Thomas.
7. McCann, M. (1978). *Health Hazards Manual for Artists*. New York: Foundation for the Community of Artists.
8. Rich, M.K. (1960). *Handcrafts for the Homebound Handicapped*. Springfield, IL: Charles C. Thomas.
9. Ayres, A.J. (1949). An analysis of crafts in the treatment of electroshock patients. *American Journal of Occupational Therapy*, 3(4), 195-198.
10. Fidler, G.S. & Fidler, J.W. (1954). *Introduction to Psychiatric Occupational Therapy*. New York: The MacMillan Co.
11. Wilkinson, V.C. & Heater, S.L. (1979). *Therapeutic Media and Techniques of Application: A Guide for Activities Therapists*. New York: Van Nostrand Reinhold Company.
12. Gould, E. & Gould, L. (1971). *Crafts for the Elderly*. Springfield, IL: Charles C. Thomas Publisher.
13. Weisberg, N. & Wilder, R. (1985). *Creative Arts With Older Adults: A Sourcebook*. New York: Human Sciences Press.

10
Mosaics

Introduction

Mosaic, which is a surface decoration made of small assembled pieces, is an ancient art form probably originating in the Middle East 5,000 years ago. Mosaics became very popular during the early Christian era perhaps because of its durability. Mosaics were used to make murals of sermons in pictures at a time when most people were unable to read. In those times, small pieces of colored glass, ceramic fragments and stone were pressed into fresh plaster or concrete. The mosaic artist would have the picture and layout, colors and shading firmly in mind. It would be necessary to do only a small area at a time and to work fast (Figure 10-1). The process used today is much easier.[1-3] Some other cultures in which mosaics are an important craft or art form are Greece, Egypt, Italy, Mexico, France, Thailand, Jordan and America.

Frequency of Use

Approximately one third of clinics use mosaics once a week and another one third use mosaics somewhat less often than one time per week. As a treatment, it is most often used to improve fine motor control or to encourage self-expression.

Assessments

Mosaic requires few tools, is not too messy and has the capability of assisting in assessing many functional areas such as size and color

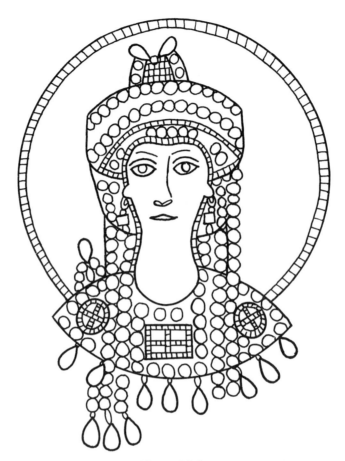

Figure 10-1
Historical Mosaic—The Empress Theodora in San Vitale, Ravenna, Italy

discrimination, ability to make decisions, fine motor skills, spatial awareness, ability to follow directions, and ability to plan and carry out a plan. It is included in many activity batteries. (Refer to Figure 6-1 for a profile of which crafts are used in each assessment.) One of the earliest in occupational therapy was the Shoemyen Diagnostic Test Battery developed between 1963 and 1967. This assessment includes clay figure modeling, sculpture carving from a composition block, finger painting and mosaics. From one to four clients can be evaluated together. The four crafts are presented and the individual client is allowed to choose the order in which to do them. Forty-five minutes are allowed for each craft. The University of Florida developed several reporting forms for the assessment.

The Goodman Battery developed in 1967 starts out with the copying of a mosaic design, as it is considered to be the most structured part of the evaluation. This is followed by spontaneous drawing, figure drawing and clay working. The protocol for this assessment is strictly structured even in areas such as seating for client and therapist, placement of materials and the pattern to copy. Cognitive and affective functioning are assessed with this battery.[4]

Barbara Hemphill, who has written two books on psychiatric occupational therapy evaluation, began to develop the BH Battery in 1973. This battery has two activity components: mosaic tiling and finger painting. The tiling activity is done first, assessing skill in organizing. A layout for the materials is provided. Clients are not given design instruction other than gluing the tiles to the board however they like.[5]

The Tiled Trivet Assessment used at the Veterans Administration Medical Center in New York is part of a prevocational evaluation. This evaluation has several structured tasks: sorting screws, arranging a colored paper pattern, alphabetizing and the Tiled Trivet Assessment. The patient is asked to replicate a tile pattern using a cardboard background.[6]

In the Comprehensive Assessment Process for assessment of clients in a group, mosaic is used in the first of three 50-minute sessions. The client can choose from four colors to complete a mosaic board design. At the second session, there are six choices for colored grout. The behaviors assessed have to do with interpersonal interactions, work skills, self-concept, self-knowledge and leisure skills. Other activities in this assessment are magazine collage, a group mural or a hypothetic group problem-solving session about landing on the moon. The group chooses one of these three activities to do at the third session. Documentation is done on a check-off sheet.[5,7]

The Perkins Tile Task, for use in psychiatry, was presented at the 1986 Great Southern Occupational Therapy Conference in Charleston, South Carolina by Vicki Perkins, OTR. Quantitative research, number of tiles used, amount of board surface covered and tile placement were related to diagnostic groups.[8]

The Nedra Gillette Battery is a purely projective test that was developed in the 1960s. It has three activities each with a different purpose: Watercolor as an unstructured task, mosaic as the structured test and the carving of a plaster vermiculite composite block as the resistive test. A scoring scale of behavior traits was used.[7,9]

The Neuropsychiatric Institute (NPI) Interest Checklist includes mosaics among its 80 activities. Patients are asked to complete the questionnaire about the level of their interest in the various activities. A discussion between patient and therapist of the completed checklist aims to assess past, present and possible future leisure choices.[10]

Treatment with Mosaics

Perhaps the attraction of this craft for today's therapist is that mosaics fit the current short hospital stays of most patients. Tile trivets, which come in a variety of shapes, are probably the most common mosaic project. The trivet frames are metal or plywood shapes into which the mosaic is set. A 6in.-square size is often used. The metal trivets purchased through craft suppliers have a Masonite board on which to mount the tile. Some clinics simply give a 6in. by 6in. board cut in the clinic for the patients. If they finish their tile project, it is then mounted in the trivet frame. In this manner, the waste that occurs when patients do not finish their project before being discharged is diminished.

In long-term facilities, residents can attempt more challenging mosaic projects such as table tops, jewel boxes, trays or picture frames. Another traditional mosaiclike process is using various colors and shapes of dried peas, beans and pasta to cover shapes and spaces to make a picture.[11,12] These make nice kitchen decorations.

Supplies and Tools

For the usual 6in. by 6in. tile trivet, the following supplies and tools are needed. (Most supplies and tools will need to be purchased from craft vendors, however tiles may be purchased more inexpensively at local tile stores that sell tiles for kitchens and bathrooms.)

Supplies
- Paper and pencil for making the design;
- An assortment of ceramic tiles in various shapes, sizes and colors;
- A 6in. by 6in., 1/8in. Masonite board;
- Tile cement or white glue;
- Grout;
- Grout coloring (optional);
- Water or grout additive;
- Grout sealer or liquid floor wax;
- Paper towels;

Tools
- Bowl for mixing;
- Ruler for measuring spaces;
- Spoon;
- Spatula;
- Tile nippers; and
- Sponge.

PROCESS
1. Show the patient a sample of a finished trivet.
2. Have the patient plan his or her own design and choose his or her tile colors. The tiles can be arranged and rearranged to fit the space until a satisfactory design is chosen.

3. If tiles need to be cut to fit, the patient should put on goggles before cutting with the tile nippers (Figure 10-2). If the patient cuts the tiles inside a paper bag, others are also protected from flying fragments.

4. Glue the pieces down individually. Remove two at a time from the design. This allows enough working space to apply one of the two individual tiles to the board without disturbing or losing the entire design. Before gluing the second tile, remove a third to provide working space. Allow space of 1/16in. to 1/8in. between the tiles. Use a ruler as a guide if necessary. This space is wide enough for the grout to be applied between the tiles. Some suggest standing a nickle or a dime between tiles to space them properly.

5. Continue gluing until design is completed. Allow the glue to dry.

6. Mix the grout according to package directions. The powdered grout and water or grout additive mixture should be the consistency of heavy cream.

7. The grout mixture is poured or scraped with the spatula onto the tiles. Use the spatula, fingers, sponge or damp paper towels to push the grout into all the crevices. Be sure to grout the board all the way to the edge. Tap the tile to allow air bubbles to escape. This prevents holes and cracks.

8. Lightly rub the excess grout off the tiles, being careful not to rub it out of the cracks.

9. Allow grout to dry slowly overnight. Place a damp cloth or paper towel over it. If cracks appear, mix another batch of grout and apply it into the cracks.

10. When the grout is completely dry, rub any remaining film of grout off the tiles.

11. Fit the tiled board into the trivet frame.

12. Apply the grout sealer. Liquid floor wax can be used as a grout sealer.[1-3,13]

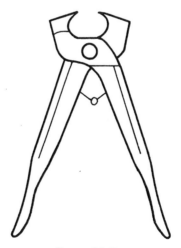

Figure 10-2
Tile Nippers

Main Therapeutic Applications

Physical Dysfunction

For the most part, fine motor coordination can be addressed through the making of mosaics by the physically disabled patient. Picking up the tiles can improve pinch. Gripping the tile nippers can be used to strengthen cylindrical grasp. The special aspects of planning and arranging the design can be important areas for those patients with brain trauma such as head injury or cerebrovascular accident.[1,14] Mosaics may be done by bed patients and those in isolation up to the point of mixing and applying grout. That process is best done near a sink that has a clay or plaster trap to prevent the grout from clogging the drain. For the bed-bound, ward-bound patients, the therapist might want to take the project to the clinic and do the grouting for them. For the one-handed patient, gluing the tile down may make this craft too difficult and frustrating. Mixing the grout and water may cause dust in the air, which would be contraindicated for respiratory patients.

Mental Health

Mosaics offer opportunities to work on problems that affect many mental health patients: attention span, concentration, planning, spacial relationship, sequencing and fine motor control. This may be why mosaics are so often used in psychiatric occupational therapy assessments. Even very-low-functioning patients can achieve a good product outcome with mosaics. By increasing the tile color and shape choice, size and complexity of the project, it is possible to grade mosaics from very easy to difficult.

Pediatrics

Pediatric patients are often working to improve fine motor performance. Mosaics provide an excellent opportunity to practice this skill. The time required to glue all the tiles frequently exceeds the attention span of many children. Gluing may need to be done in several sessions. Another inexpensive possibility with children is to use seeds and beans. Simply cover each individual section with glue and scatter the seeds on that section. Shake off the excess onto a newspaper and pour the excess back into the seed container. This speeds up the process for children's shorter attention spans. Another adaptation of mosaics for children is paper mosaics. A variety of shapes, sizes and colors of construction paper are used to make a design that can be glued to cardboard or paper. Girls sometimes enjoy sedentary mosaic activity more than boys.

Geriatrics

Adaptation of mosaics for the elderly may include using the 3/4in. tiles rather than the 3/8in. size. This increases the tiles' visibility and the ease with which they are handled. The therapist may choose highly contrasting colors as these also make them more visible. If white or light tiles are glued on the dark brown Masonite, they show up well. Mosaic materials are usually not breakable. This is beneficial as many elderly patients have poor balance, which makes it difficult for them to walk and to get in and out of chairs, which may cause them to drop things. They may lack the grip strength to use the tile nippers. The trivet project usually takes not longer than three sessions, thus sustaining their interest. This simple yet attractive craft can be appealing to the elderly as its rich history can make it seem like a prestigious craft and thus age appropriate.

Case Study

Michael is a 69-year-old Lebanese immigrant. He grew up in Beirut in a Christian family. After attending a school run by missionaries, he went to France to study architecture at a university. World War Two broke out while he was in France. He joined the French Army, was captured and spent several years as a prisoner of war. After the war, he returned to Beirut and completed his architectural studies at the American University. Michael joined an architectural company and began to develop a name for himself locally as a restoration specialist for old buildings. In 1950 his family assisted him in arranging a marriage with a second cousin. The couple had four children during the next ten years.

He and his wife were very concerned about their children's education. They sacrificed luxuries to send their children to private schools and to the university. As the three older children finished college, they left the parental home. The eldest, a girl, followed in her father's footsteps and went to France to study medicine. The second eldest, a male, took a job working in Saudi Arabia. The next boy was accepted as a student at the University of Oklahoma and went to the United States, leaving only the youngest daughter at home. The three children living in other countries returned home for yearly visits.

When Israel invaded Lebanon, Michael and his wife and daughter remained in their home which Michael had built gradually in stages over the years in the Christian section of Beirut. As the war progressed and the bombing came closer, the three older children began to press their parents to emigrate. In 1984, Michael's wife died of a heart attack during a particularly close and heavy bomb attack. At last, he was persuaded to emigrate to the United States where his youngest son lived with his American wife.

He and the youngest daughter, who was 25 years old, were crowded into this American home. Michael had to share a room with his grandson. Shortly after his arrival, he began to have angina. The physician who examined him found him to be a good candidate for open heart surgery for coronary artery disease. This was performed in 1985. Following this surgery, Michael became very fearful and depressed. He became a cardiac cripple, refusing to do the exercises advised by his physician. He just sat on the sofa in front of the television. He then developed a sleep disturbance, sleep apnea. The combination of the sleep problem with the inactivity caused him to become increasingly depressed and cranky. His son's family found him to be very disturbing to their family life. His daughter, who spoke very little English, was of little help in coping with her father. When he began to refuse to eat, his condition rapidly deteriorated.

Finally, he had a panic attack, fearing he was dying. His son called the ambulance. He was taken to the emergency department. After a triage screening, it was decided he needed further observation for his disorientation but not for his heart. He was admitted to the geropsychiatric unit of the hospital. His physician consulted with the psychiatrist on the unit and they gave him a diagnosis of organic anxiety syndrome with depression and sleep apnea. Both physicians advised gradually increasing his activity level while they ran further tests.

The occupational therapist evaluated Michael using a geriatric sensory screening and The Goodman Battery. On the mosaic tile task, he surprised the therapist by completing the replication of the tile sample quickly and accurately. He mentioned that some of the buildings he had restored in Beirut had had mosaic floor tiles. His spontaneous drawing was a sketch of one of the buildings Michael remembered working on years ago. In the human figure drawings, he drew a typical Middle Eastern workman holding a shovel and wearing the traditional Arab headdress. He said he was too tired to finish the clay portion of the test that day, so it was postponed. His physicians at this time discovered he had an obstructed airway. Surgery was performed to remove the obstruction. The occupational therapist went to visit him in the recovery room. When he returned to the geropsychiatric unit the next day, she showed him some books on mosaics that she had checked out of the public library. She set a book rack up for him on his bedside table and stayed with him for one half hour while he looked at books and discussed them. He never finished the clay portion of The Goodman Battery because he became involved in creating a mosaic table top to give to his daughter-in-law. As he began to eat and sleep better and to draw his mosaic design and choose his tiles, his depression began to lift and the dementia seemed to clear. He completed the mosaic design but was unable to finish putting on the legs before his discharge. Before he was discharged, the COTA took Michael to a local senior center to orient him to resources for senior citizens. Initially he was reluctant and shy, as he was the only male with 15 women at the center.

The activity director assured Michael that there were several other men who attended, too. He appeared pleased and mildly excited by the arts and crafts area and the prospect of finishing his table.

Discussion Questions

1. Would one of the other assessment batteries have been a better choice for Michael? Why?
2. If Michael had been dissatisfied with the ceramic mosaic tiles available to him in the occupational therapy clinic, what could the therapist have done to get glass tiles, which were satisfactory to him? Where might a therapist go to find glass tiles that are seldom used now rather than the ceramic tiles she had available?
3. What precautions could be necessary for a patient who just had an airway obstruction removed?

References

1. Department of the Army. (1971). *Craft Techniques in Occupational Therapy.* Washington DC: US Government Printing Office.
2. Moseley, S., Johnson, P., & Koenig, H. (1962). *Crafts Design.* Belmont, CA: Wadsworth.
3. Reader's Digest. (1979). *Crafts and Hobbies.* Pleasantville, NY: The Reader's Digest Association Inc.
4. Hemphill, B.J. (1982a). *The Evaluative Process in Psychiatric Occupational Therapy.* Thorofare, NJ: Slack.
5. Hemphill, B.J. (1982b). *Training Manual for the BH Battery.* Thorofare, NJ: Slack.
6. Jacobs, K. (1985). *Occupational Therapy: Work-Related Programs and Assessments.* Boston: Little, Brown.
7. Practice Division. (1985). *Computers: Information Packet.* Rockville, MD: American Occupational Therapy Association.
8. Perkins, V.J. (1986). Quantitative assessment of a mosaic tile task. *Abstracts of the Fourth Annual Meeting.* The Great Southern Occupational Therapy Conference. Charleston, South Carolina.
9. Gillette, N. (July 12, 1989). Personal communication—Telephone interview and letter regarding Nedra Gillette's Battery. Birmingham, AL.
10. Matsutsuya, J.S. (1969). The interest checklist. *American Journal of Occupational Therapy,* 24(4).
11. Better Homes and Gardens. (1966). *Stitchery and Crafts.* New York: Meredith Press.
12. Janitch, V. (1973). *Country Crafts.* New York: Viking Press.
13. VanZandt, E. (1973). *Crafts for Fun and Profit.* London: Aldus Books.
14. Overs, R.P., O'Conner, E., & Demarco, B. (1974). *Avocational Activities for the Handicapped.* Springfield, IL: Charles C. Thomas.

11
Ceramics

▬▬▬▬
▼

Introduction

The ancient craft of ceramics involves simply shaping clay, an especially plastic earth, allowing it to dry, and then baking it at a high temperature for a long time. Ceramics may be one of our oldest crafts developed after leatherworking and woodworking. We know humans have been shaping clay and baking it for 10,000 years. In fact, the durability of pottery fragments have made it possible for archeologists to learn much about prehistoric humans. On the other hand, ceramics break, so intact ancient pieces are rare. These characteristics, brittleness and durability, remain, despite our advanced technology in other areas.[1]

Ceramics is an encompassing term that includes pottery, ceramic sculpture, ceramic tiles used in kitchens and bathrooms, ceramic building blocks and decorative facades for buildings, beads and jewelry as well as the ceramic tiles used to protect the bodies of space shuttles. The scope of this book includes only a minute part of what are called ceramics—only those objects usually made by patients working with occupational therapists: smaller pots, sculptures and jewelry.

Frequency of Use

One quarter to one third of therapists use ceramics in their clinical practice. The most frequently used types are slip-molded greenware and ceramic sculpture. Few clinics and therapists are able to afford the time and energy expenditure to use the potter's wheel. However, since ceramics techniques are similar to those of a variety of less durable shaping and sculpting materials, it was thought best to present these basic craft techniques, which can be adapted to the other materials.

Assessments

Standardized occupational therapy assessments that use clay as part of a complete evaluation are The Goodman Battery, The Shoemyen Battery, The Azima Battery, Carolyn Owens Activity Battery, Gillette's Battery, Nelson Clark's Clay Test, Androes, Dreyfus and Bloesch Diagnostic Occupational Therapy Test Battery, Gross Activity Battery, and O'Kane Diagnostic Battery. These are all evaluations used with psychiatric patients. In most of them, the patient is asked to use the clay provided to make something. However the Shoemyen Battery specifically asks the patient to model a human figure.[2] Each of these evaluations includes the projective clay sculpture as part of a battery of activities. Even Clark's Clay Test is part of the Clark Battery.[3] Clay is included because it is a part of natural human development to attempt to shape. Scribbling and drawing have similar developmental sequences. Initially, the child smears, feels and squeezes clay and then molds shapes.[4,5] Clay is viewed as the most unstructured of all projective assessments[2] because of the effort needed to control it. Its plastic quality allows a patient to make a mistake and reverse it. The aspects of clay that allow a patient to express many emotions, ideas and qualities also cause difficulty for those with perceptual dysfunction.[2] Three-dimensional media are more difficult to conceptualize than two-dimensional media for purposes of construction.[6]

Supplies

It is possible to use ceramics in a room or section off the occupational therapy clinic following safety guidelines for kiln wiring and venting. Such specifications are usually available through the safety officer of your hospital or clinic or the local ceramics store. The sink for ceramics needs to have a clay sediment trap in the drainpipe to allow clay residue to be easily removed and thus avoid costly plumbing bills. The following supplies and equipment are sufficient for most clinic ceramics and for the techniques discussed in this book, although more sophisticated materials and techniques are available.

Supplies:
- Ready-mixed clay;
- Ready-mixed slip;
- Ready-mixed glazes;
- Bisque stains and spray;
- Fine-grain sponges;
- Pyrometric cones;

- Kiln wash; and
- Underglazes.

Tools and equipment:

- Covered plastic clay storage container;
- Storage shelves;
- Kiln;
- Kiln furniture;
- Stilts;
- Canvas-covered boards;
- Clay pull (cutting wire);
- Fettling knife;
- Sgraffito/cleaning tool;
- Needle tool;
- Wire-loop tool;
- Rolling pin;
- Plaster or masonite bats;
- Slip molds;
- Slip strainer;
- Mold straps;
- Sink;
- Plastic water bowls; and
- Glaze brushes.

Process

Most therapists buy ready-ground and mixed clay as the preparation is difficult and requires extensive costly machinery. Clay is usually purchased in 25-pound plastic bags that measure approximately 14in. by 5in. by 5in. Clay comes in a variety of grays, browns and reds. Clay can have grog added, which is previously fired clay ground up like sand. This adds strength to the clay but is contraindicated for many patients as it can be abrasive to the hands. Different clays may fire at different temperatures, however, most occupational therapists simplify their ceramics operation by firing at only one or two temperatures, usually between 1,800 degrees and 2,000 degrees Fahrenheit or 980 degrees and 1,100 degrees centigrade. The first step in preparing the ready-mixed clay is to cut and form it into usable 3in. to 4in. diameter pieces. This is most easily accomplished by using the clay pull, which is a tool one can easily make by cutting a 20in. length of thin wire or nylon fishing line and tying each end to a large button or bead.

The clay pull is grasped at each end and wound around the fingers until it is quite close to the clay. The line is laid across the block and pressed straight down through the clay until the proper size piece can be pulled off. This piece is then wedged. Professional ceramicists wedge clay in a kneading pattern but in occupational therapy the most common method is to throw the clay onto a wedging board as shown in the illustration (Figure 11-1). The purpose of wedging is to redistribute the moisture equally to make the clay softer and easier to handle and to get rid of any air pockets that could possibly cause the piece to explode in the kiln as the heated air expands during firing. The wedged clay is then cut on a wire (Figure 11-2) or with the clay pull to assure that no air pockets remain (Figure 11-3). It is then rewedged before using.

There are six basic methods of forming ceramics in occupational therapy. They are described and illustrated sequentially below from the easiest technique, pinch pots, to the most difficult and exacting, the potter's wheel.

Pinch Pot

PROCESS
1. Form the clay into a ball.
2. Stick the thumb into the top of the ball. This makes the first opening.
3. With the thumb of the dominant hand on the inside and fingers on the outside, begin to press gently out with the thumb moving the form either clockwise or counter clockwise while keeping the piece supported with the nondominant hand (Figure 11-4).

    Continue to move the beginning vessel in this fashion until the walls and bottom are uniformly 1/2in. thick or less. If small cracks appear on the edge near the opening, just pinch them together.
4. Set the pot on a canvas-covered board and using both hands, smooth the walls. Do not use water to smooth the walls at this point, as it will weaken them.
5. Set the pot aside to dry on a mesh shelf or grate so air can reach all surfaces.

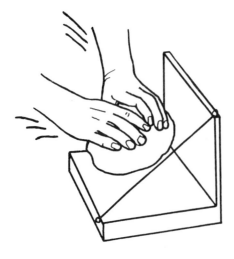

Figure 11-1
Wedging on a Wedging Board

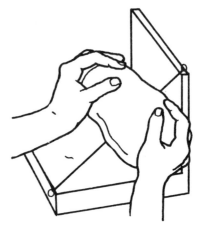

Figure 11-2
Cutting Clay on the Wire

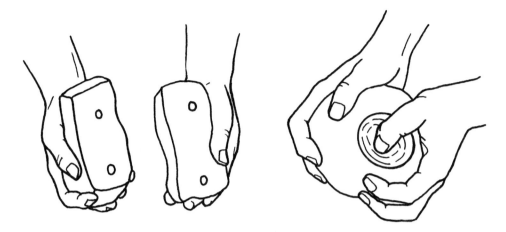

Figure 11-3
Air Pockets in Unwedged Clay

Figure 11-4
Pinch Pot

6. After it is leather hard, which is the hardness of good shoe leather, smooth the pot with a damp, fine-grain sponge. At this stage, carve or incise the surface for decoration.

   The length of the drying process depends on the temperature, humidity and movement of the air. Most hospitals have a fairly dry atmosphere. Therapists will need to experiment to find how long it takes a piece to dry to bone dry, which is when the piece is not cool to the touch, but feels like room temperature. Then the piece will be ready to bisque fire, a process to be described later.

Slab Building

Slab construction is the next most complicated process.

PROCESS

1. On a canvas-covered board, roll the wedged clay with a rolling pin to an even thickness of 1/2in. to 1/4in.
2. Lay a previously made paper pattern on the clay. Cut around the pattern with a fettling knife (Figure 11-5), a special clay tool for cutting.
3. After a short time in which pieces are allowed to stiffen slightly, join the pieces in the following manner. Lift the base off the canvas and place it on a plaster bat.
4. Incise or score all the edges that are to be joined by using a tool called a needle, which is a wooden cylinder handle with a 1-1/2in. pin stuck into the end (Figure 11-6). The incising should be in a crosshatch manner. Each seam will have two crosshatch edges.
5. Moisten both edges with finger before pressing them together. This moisture goes into the incisions and makes a

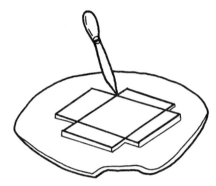

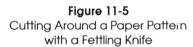

Figure 11-5
Cutting Around a Paper Pattern
with a Fettling Knife

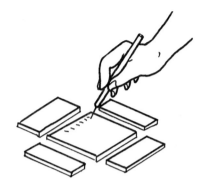

Figure 11-6
Crosshatching with a Clay Needle

natural slip. Slip is a liquid clay that is used for a variety of purposes, one of which will be described later. In slab building, one must be careful not to allow the clay to become too wet, as that weakens the structure.

6. Strengthen the joints by pressing a coil of clay on the interior surface and smoothing it into the walls.
7. Then set the piece aside until leather hard, when it can be decorated by sgrafitto or textured with a comb or by making impressions with buttons or other small objects.

Slab building may offer the most variety of all techniques in ceramics. Napkin rings can be constructed with one simple joint. A simple slab scored on the bottom to prevent warping and decorated with surface designs makes an attractive trivet. A draped slab can be made by laying a trimmed clay slab over another object to dry. Buttons, buckles and windchime parts can all be cut from a plain slab.

Coil Building
Coil building is an elaboration of the slab-building technique.

PROCESS
1. Make a round or oval base slab (Figure 11-7).
2. Score or incise the edge where the coil will be placed.
3. Make the coils by rolling the piece back and forth with both hands on the canvas covered board (Figure 11-8).
4. Wet the scored edge and lay the coil on it.
5. Press it lightly to bond the two pieces.
6. Lightly moisten the top of the coil; lay another coil on this seam and lightly press.

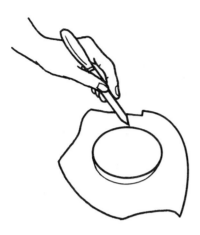

Figure 11-7
Cutting a Round Base for a Coil Pot

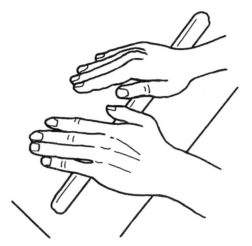

Figure 11-8
Coils Being Made

7. Continue this process until the desired height is reached. If the pot is to curve outward, set the coil a little to the outside of the one below it. If it is to curve inward, place the coil a little toward the inside top surface of the preceding coil.

8. When the desired shape and size are reached, smooth the sides. Many people like the look of coil pots and, consequently, do nothing to change the surface. It is possible to use coils in making the base, but these are never quite as strong as a slab base. In each slip-bonded joint lies the potential for weakness and possible cracking.

9. Another easy coil method, especially for wide, low bowls, which might collapse of their own weight while damp, is to select a ready-made bowl, line it with plastic wrap, lay the slab for the base in the bottom of the bowl and then lay the coils up the sides of the bowl. A design can be made with the coils (Figure 11-9). The plastic wrap leaves hardly any marks.

10. Coils should be smoothed on the inside of the bowl to fasten them together, for neatness and easy washability.

11. The coiled bowl should be left inside the ready-made bowl until it is leather-hard and it can be lifted out.

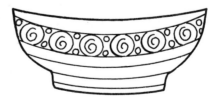

Figure 11-9
A Bowl With Coil Design

Sculpture

Sculpture in occupational therapy is often an activity in which the therapist offers very little instruction or direction to the patient. Sculpture incorporates the techniques used to make pinch pots, slab containers and coil vessels as well as techniques not previously mentioned. One such technique involves using a piece of clay and hollowing the center out by using a wire loop tool to systematically cut away pieces of clay from the middle or inside of a bulky sculpture. This prevents an explosion as sculptures with thick walls are prone to blow up in the kiln. Another technique is to use a paper core or substructure and form the clay sculpture around it. The paper core, which supports the sculpture's walls and keeps it from collapsing in on itself, will burn away in the kiln, leaving a hollow sculpture. Professional sculptors use other techniques in building larger, more complex figures but they are too involved for most clinic situations. Children often assemble parts when making a sculpture, for example, sticking a head, arms, and legs to a torso to make a person. These parts often break off in handling or firing unless the child uses the correct technique for joining parts.

Slip Casting

Slip casting is often used by many therapists because of the chances of a successful product, which will please the patient and increase self-esteem.

Mold making is a complex process requiring skills beyond the scope of this book. Many moderately priced molds are available at local ceramic hobby stores.

PROCESS

1. First check the slip-casting molds for cleanliness and gently wipe them out with a damp sponge or fine bristle paint brush, if necessary, to remove old clay.
2. Fit the mold sections together and fasten them tightly with mold straps or giant rubber bands.
3. Mix and strain the slip to remove any lumps.
4. Pour the slip into the mold pour spout (Figure 11-10) to the top.
5. As the plaster absorbs moisture from the slip, it will sink down in the pour spout. It is necessary to check the mold every few minutes and to refill it to the top.
6. When the thickness of the solid clay near the plaster becomes approximately 1/4in., pour out the remainder of the slip by turning the mold over to drain (Figure 11-11). This slip can be saved and reused if stored properly in an airtight container.
7. After approximately 1/2 hour, turn the mold upright and carefully remove one half of the mold.
8. Cut off the excess clay in the pour spout. The piece can

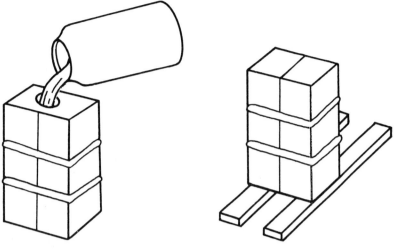

Figure 11-10
Pouring Slip into a Mold

Figure 11-11
Draining the Mold

remain in the half mold until it becomes leather hard. It will then easily come out of the mold, because in drying it will shrink away from the plaster (Figure 11-12).

9. If the slip casting mold has textured walls, allow it to dry before cleaning the seams with a sgraffito/cleaning tool. If the slip cast mold has no texture or detail, the seam can be removed at the leather-hard stage with a fine-grain sponge. There are a variety of other molds, press molds and drape molds that can also be used with regular clay instead of slip. These molds are usually one piece into which clay is pressed or draped and removed when leather-hard.

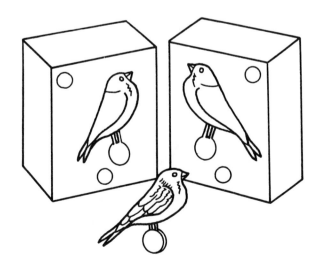

Figure 11-12
Removing Piece from the Mold

Pottery Wheel

Throwing on the potter's wheel is one of the most sophisticated ceramic techniques. Consequently, few clinics use it because of the skill required for a patient to create an object successfully. Only the most basic steps will be given here. Students of ceramics wishing for more information will find a variety of source books.[6-10]

PROCESS

1. Experiment with the foot pedal or switch to determine how much pressure or power is required to achieve desired speed.
2. Affix a bat on the center of the wheel. A bowl of water and a sponge should be nearby.
3. Very slightly dampen the bat.
4. Place a ball of wedged clay the size of an orange onto the center of the bat (Figure 11-13).
5. Start the wheel slowly and check with a finger to be sure the ball is in the center of the wheel. If it is not, stop the wheel and reposition the clay. Repeat this until the ball is as close as possible to the center. Then with the wheel stopped, press it down to fasten it to the bat.
6. The clay must be kept "slippery" wet so that it slips through the hands. The potter needs to constantly reapply water to the surface. The wheel should always be moving before the hands touch the clay and be kept moving after the hands have been gently removed from the clay. Begin to spin the wheel and press the palms of both hands down and around the base of the clay to center it (Figure 11-14). Keeping the forearms braced on the thighs helps stabilize the hands and wrists. The basic principle to remember is that force to the clay should be transmitted through pressure

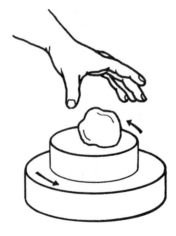

Figure 11-13
Tossing Clay onto the Center of the Bat

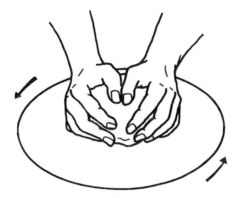

Figure 11-14
Centering the Clay

from the large bones of the arm and wrist so the muscles don't cramp and tire and because it works better.

7. Coning is the next step in which the clay is actually mixed by pressing to raise it to a cone then steadily pressing down on the top of the cone with the right hand while supporting the clay with the left hand (Figure 11-15). This is all done with the palms of the hands, not the fingers. In occupational therapy, patients are encouraged to practice joint protection using large muscles and joints rather than putting stress on the more vulnerable small joints and tendons. Advanced potters repeat the coning process several times before the next step (Figure 11-16). Beginners may omit coning and move immediately to step 8.

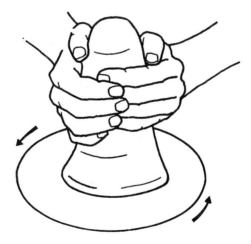

Figure 11-15
Coning the Clay

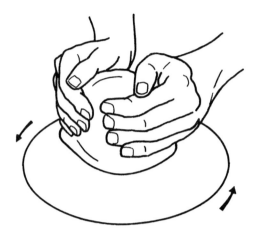

Figure 11-16
Pressing Down on Clay in Preparation for Reconing

8. Open the clay. This is achieved by pressing the right thumb into the middle of centered clay as the wheel continues to move. The thumb is pressed to a depth that leaves about 1in. of clay between the thumb and the bat. Then place both thumbs in the hole and begin to widen the hole slowly and gently until the floor of the pot is the desired width (Figure 11-17).

9. Next, raise the walls by interlocking the thumbs and placing the fingers of the left hand inside the hole and the right on the outside. As the wheel revolves, apply gentle pressure while pulling up at the same time. Keeping the elbows in at the side or with forearms on the thighs improves control. Repeat this motion until the desired height is reached. For beginners,

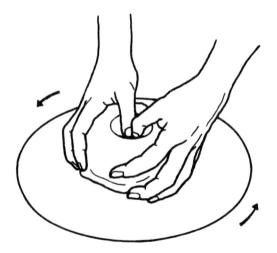

Figure 11-17
Opening Up the Clay

objects of 6in. in height and 4in. in diameter are all that should be attempted. Simple cylinders or bowls are adequate for most patients. Shaping the clay into other than a cylindrical shape or small bowl takes skill and practice.

10. When the pot is fully formed, use a damp sponge to smooth the inside of the pot and absorb excess water, which could weaken the walls.

11. Level the top of the vessel by placing the needle tool through the wall 1/2in. or 1/4in. below the top while the wheel is turning slowly and trimming away this clay until the top edge is even. Then smooth the rim with wet fingers or a sponge while the wheel is turning.

12. Loosen the vessel by pulling the clay pull between the pot and the masonite bat once. This is not necessary with plaster bats.

13. Then set the pot aside on the bat until leather hard.

14. Lift the pot off the bat.

15. Turn it upside down, center it on the wheel and stabilize it with three pieces of fresh clay. This process, called turning, involves trimming off the excess clay at the base.

16. Make concentric circles with the needle tool while the wheel turns (Figure 11-18).

17. Then, pare the excess clay by using cutting tools. Take the pot off the bat.

18. Texture or incise the walls for decoration and allow the pot to dry.

Firing the Kiln

Each kiln comes with a firing manual that gives a timing guide and loading directions. Most clinic firing is between the pyrometric cone

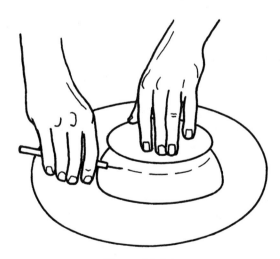

Figure 11-18
Trimming the Pot With the Needle Tool

range of 07 to 03. The first firing is called the bisque firing, which causes the clay to harden enough so that it will not disintegrate if it becomes wet. For patients all clay should be bisque fired to make the piece more durable before glaze is applied.

Glazes

Glazes in clinics are almost always ready-mixed as some of the ingredients when in the dry state are hazardous to health. Commercial glazes have specific directions for application and firing temperature on the label. Glazes should dry at least six hours before firing.

Underglazes. Underglaze is another kind of surface decoration. It can be brushed, sponged, spattered or sprayed onto bisqueware. Look at the label for application and firing instructions. Then the piece must be fired again before applying clear or semitransparent overglaze. Underglazed pieces need an overglaze and a third firing to give a water impermeable surface. Underglaze offers opportunities for experimentation such as brushing the underglaze into incisions on the surface to emphasize them, or brushing the underglaze over a textured surface and rubbing away some of the glaze to emphasize the texture. Ceramic hobbyists often brush underglaze onto greenware but greenware is usually too fragile for most sick people to handle with the delicacy required. It is necessary to bisque fire everything in the clinic before glazing or underglazing.

Bisque Stains. For purely decorative pieces such as figurines and some kinds of jewelry, bisque stains can be painted on the surface. These stains, which are unfired, are not moisture resistant and cannot be used in any container for liquids. However, they have some qualities that make them useful in the clinic.

They do not require as much time or as many processes as traditional glazes. They are applied in much the same way as liquid tempra paints would be and like tempra colors, need to have a protective finish over them. Most commonly, a spray sealer is used. This kind of sealer needs to be applied where there is adequate ventilation, preferably outdoors. In some situations, the patient can apply the stain to the bisqueware and the therapist will then apply the lacquer sealer for the patient. Be careful to avoid setting the piece with those to be fired as they may be hard to tell apart at firing time.

The last firing is the glaze firing. Glazed pieces should be set on stilts and placed so there is at least 1/2in. between each piece and the walls. This allows air to circulate thus avoiding spotty glazes. Patients, like many ceramicists, have difficulty waiting the length of time required for proper kiln cooling. A rule of thumb is to let the kiln cool twice as long as it took to fire it to full temperature. This will avoid having glazes craze and crackle from cooling too fast.

Main Therapeutic Applications

Physical Dysfunction

In the past, before the age of therapy putty, ceramic clay was used to achieve all the same benefits for which that expensive medium is now used. Squeezing, pushing, pinching, patting, rolling, smoothing and manipulating clay can achieve almost any wrist, hand or finger movement desired. Working with clay strengthens the upper extremities and can easily be graded from the delicate manipulations such as patting, to pushing, to pressing, to throwing clay during wedging or wedging by kneading. Wedging can achieve shoulder flexion and extension. Rolling the clay uses the abdominals, elbow extensors and flexors. The therapist must be careful that the table and chair are the proper height to achieve the desired movement. Positioning of the project will define which muscles are used. The therapist needs to think through exactly which motions are desired and raise and lower the project, place it close or far or to the side of the patient to achieve the desired movement. Fine motor control and coordination can be enhanced by scoring the clay in slab or coil building, or surface decorative techniques such as sgraffito or painting with underglazes.

Theoretically, the kick wheel should be good for strengthening knee extensors, but practically, throwing a pot on the wheel requires so much concentration and skill that it is difficult to coordinate the upper extremity with the needs of a healing lower extremity. Clay can be used with bedside patients as it is noise free if the clay is already wedged. Damp clay is nontoxic and easily washable. It can be worked with or without tools. All these attributes make it a good medium to carry into the room of a patient confined for infectious disease. It is less expensive than therapy putty and can be left in the patient's room. A masonite square covered with paper can be used as a work surface. If an infectious patient completes a project for firing, the whole working surface with clay on top can be put into a plastic bag to be carried to the kiln. All infectious agents will be killed in firing. The paper should be bagged for disposal like all other infection controlled materials. The masonite can be sterilized by washing with antibacterial soap.

Clay is particularly suited for use with the blind and partially sighted because of its tactile qualities. The blind person can feel a sample and use that shape to formulate an idea to work toward. One-handed patients can succeed at coil-built pots if the therapist cuts a base. Both using the rolling pin and rolling coils can cause the patient to use a weak hand to assist or stabilize in the movement. Additionally these two movements require the patient to work on trunk control, which is a problem for many stroke patients. For patients with poor coordination, the draped slab method may achieve the best results.

Burn patients with completely healed wounds can work on decreasing contractures by working with clay. Because their skin is so tender and clay dries it out, each session with clay should be followed by using hand lotion.

Conditions in which ceramics are contraindicated are in patients whose hands have open wounds because of the possibility of infection or further damage to the wounded surface; arthritic joints can be further damaged by too much force since many ceramic techniques can stress joints; patients with circulation problems as in diabetes as even smooth clay can abrade the skin surface; patients with nerve deficits can injure their hands without feeling it.[7,11-13]

Mental Health

The opportunity for expression of thought and mood are perhaps the most beneficial aspects of clay for psychiatric patients. Listed earlier in this chapter are several psychiatric occupational therapy evaluations that use clay. The clay project can demonstrate cognitive deficits such as confusion, inability to follow instructions, and additionally, a depressed mood or bizarre thoughts. For patients with cognitive deficits, having a variety of samples for them to examine assists in conceptualizing the clay process. While schizophrenics may have difficulty with the formlessness of a pinch pot or clay sculpture, both wedging and rolling slabs or coils can achieve the shoulder external rotation and elbow extension that are so often deficient. Structured slab and coil construction can help with the sensory integration for adult psychiatric patients.[14]

Psychiatric patients may find it beneficial to make a clay symbol of a person toward whom they feel hostile and then destroy it. Breaking up old dried clay or broken projects of previously discharged patients could be used to achieve a similar goal. In the past therapists have sometimes felt that wedging or pounding clay helped release aggressive hostility; however for some patients it may cause the aggression to go to a higher level. The therapist must be very vigilant if using clay with hostile patients as many clay tools can also become weapons.

Pediatrics

Clay is a natural medium for children. They play in their food, squeezing and manipulating it in the same way they handle clay. They make mud pies. Clay allows this same kind of unstructured exploration of materials. Many theorists have associated clay with the anal phase in Freud's psychosexual stages as its texture, color and consistency resemble feces.[15]

Children's competency in drawing will be reflected in how they manipulate clay and clay tools. Those who have had little experience in working with art materials or tools usually will not work as long or as independently with clay. They will often produce an unrecognizable lump and move on to more familiar activities. As children show more maturity, they will often name the lump even though it may still be unrecognizable. Gradually, children will begin to make a head which is separate from the body and add facial features, progressing in the same developmental way they do in drawing. Preadolescent children try to make realistic objects. Younger children may be less intentional about making a permanent object. They are usually more willing to put their clay back into the container after they have satisfied their curiosity and creative urge. Older children and adolescents more often feel strongly about having their objects fired and eventually glazed. While even young children may want the piece fired, they may not care about glazing it.[16] Clay is a common ingredient in play therapy situations. It fits well with the permissiveness of this kind of pediatric treatment. It allows for smearing and the messiness associated with clay and children.[17]

Children who have never been allowed to be messy or who have been punished for getting dirty or soiling themselves may have difficulty initially. Eventually most children are able to overcome this sort of anxiety and experience the pure sensual joy of wet clay. The main precautions with this population are ingestion of the materials and while clay is usually not toxic, glazes are very dangerous and best avoided with small children unless closely supervised. Children tend to make small objects with many appendages such as legs for animals. They almost always break off either before or during firing but can be glued together after firing. If the child has used a mainly two-dimensional scheme, the fired clay can be glued to paper and painted rather than glazed. Many therapists allow children to paint their bisque-fired clay objects with tempera paints rather than glazes. The washability of clay materials also make them a good choice for pediatric bedside therapy.

Geriatrics

Many of the same indicators for therapeutic use of ceramics in physical dysfunction apply to the elderly. In using clay with older people, it is best to start out with simple hand-built projects rather than molds as it is hard to wean them away from molds once they have started. Molds place fewer requirements for creativity and experimentation. However, slip-molded green ware may be a way to entice a regressed elder to begin to participate again in activities. They need to be reminded that the process of making something is more important than a beautiful final product.[18] Because so many elderly people have joint limitations it is important to help them compensate for this by positioning their projects closer to their bodies.

Elderly people often have sensory loss such as vision, hearing and tactile perception. Clay for the visually impaired may provide a creative experience they could not have with something more exacting like needlework. Hearing-impaired patients may be unaware of disturbing another patient when wedging as they don't hear the noise they are making. People with tactile deficits are in danger of injuring themselves and remaining unaware of the injury. Clay can be incorporated into a memory group by asking "What does this remind you of?" Such a question will elicit a variety of responses from elders.

Case Study

A 26-year-old married white female was admitted to a 20-bed inpatient psychiatric unit in a small private community hospital. Her diagnosis was major depression. Jean and her husband had recently moved to the city from a smaller city where her family lived. She had left her elementary teaching job to follow her engineer husband whose company had transferred him to a nearby plant. Her symptoms were loss of appetite; weight loss; early morning awakening; complaints of sleeplessness, fatigue, decreased attention span, delusional thinking related to contamination of canned and frozen foods, agoraphobia, and suicidal thoughts without concrete plan for accomplishment. The occupational therapist used the Comprehensive Occupational Therapy Evaluation Scale. She included the patient in a tissue paper flower-making group and observed her during this session. Jean showed mild to moderate dysfunction in all areas except appearance and reality orientation, which were normal. The therapist set goals to increase activity level and increase self-esteem through continued craft group involvement.

The second day Jean and one other patient were the only ones attending the occupational therapy craft group. The therapist presented a variety of craft options to the patients. Jean was unable to make a choice so the therapist gave her a grapefruit-sized ball of gray clay. She at first seemed unable to decide how to start forming the clay though she mentioned having used clay with her elementary school students. After several self-deprecatory statements about her inability to do anything good, she began to stroke the clay and manipulate it. By the end of the 1 1/2-hour occupational therapy craft session, she had formed a seal on a rock (Figure 11-19). The therapists helped her cover it with plastic so it would not dry out and so she could work on it the next day. At the next session, she used a wire loop tool to hollow out the rock and give it some facets. Two days later on Friday, it was dry enough to fire along with the projects of several other patients. The patient had worked on more paper flowers to decorate her new home on those intervening days. Over the weekend the kiln cooled down and on Monday, the patient appeared to be lying in wait for the therapist to open the kiln. Her medication had been working, the nursing staff reported. She was much more animated.

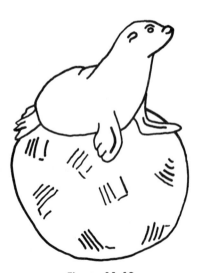

Figure 11-19
Seal on a Rock

The therapist had warned her as she opened the kiln of the possibility that her seal might have exploded in the kiln because of the thickness of its body. Fortunately, the piece fired well. Jean smiled excitedly when she saw her white bisque-fired seal. She immediately began to select glazes. She chose a glossy black for the seal and a matte green for the rock. That day her physician, with the treatment team, decided she was well enough and stabilized on her medication to be discharged. After she packed, she came to the occupational therapist and asked how she would be able to get her seal. The occupational therapist told her she could come by on Thursday to pick it up as she would be firing the kiln again on Wednesday. When she came to pick it up, she was dressed for a teaching job interview. Jean sat down with the OT and discussed why she had made the seal. She said she felt like she was stuck out on the rock all alone away from her family and long-time friends. She said she felt that now she was able to get down off the rock and begin to swim again.

The job interview was symbolic of her willingness to face life again. She thanked the therapist and said she'd like to visit again but she never did. Later the occupational therapist heard from the psychiatrist that Jean had taken a job in a suburban school and was doing well.

Discussion Questions

1. Would you have done anything differently with Jean? If so, what?
2. What kinds of patients might be bothered by the dust from cleaning a seam with a sgraffito tool on a slip-molded object?
3. Do males or females identify more with ceramics? How might this affect their participation? What could you do to get someone to participate who thought clay was something done by the opposite sex?
4. Teenage girls often pay a great deal of attention to beautifying themselves. How could ceramics be used to take advantage of this natural developmental focus?
5. If you used the following questions with patients what answers might you get when talking with them about their ceramic projects?
   - Were you surprised at the results?
   - Were you able to let go and really work with the clay?
   - What have you learned about yourself?
   - Does this have any bearing on how you handle everyday problems?

References

1. Budworth, D.W. (1970). *An Introduction to Ceramic Science.* New York: Pergamon Press.
2. Hemphill, B.J. (1982). *The Evaluative Process in Psychiatric Occupational Therapy.* Thorofare, NJ: Slack.

3. Moyer, B. (1983). *Index of Assessments Used by Occupational Therapists in Mental Health*. Monograph. Rockville, MD: American Occupational Therapy Association.

4. Harris, D.B. (1963). *Children's Drawings as Measures of Intellectual Maturity*. New York: Harcourt, Brace and World Inc.

5. O'Kane, C.P. (1968). *The Development of a Projective Technique for Use in Psychiatric Occupational Therapy*. Buffalo: State University of New York.

6. Turoff, M.P. (1949). *How to Make Pottery and Other Ceramic Ware*. New York: Crown Publishers.

7. Department of the Army. (1980). *Craft Techniques in Occupational Therapy*. Washington DC: US Government Printing Office.

8. Hamilton, D. (1974). *The Thames and Hudson Manual of Pottery and Ceramics*. London: Thames and Hudson Ltd.

9. Nelson, G.C. (1966). *Ceramics: A Potter's Handbook*, 2nd ed. New York: Holt, Rinehart and Winston.

10. Wettlaufer, G. & Wettlaufer, N. (1976). *Getting Into Pots: A Basic Pottery Manual*. Englewood Cliffs, NJ: Prentice Hall.

11. Hamill, C.M. & Oliver, R.C. (1989). *Therapeutic Activity for the Handicapped Elderly*. Gaithersburg, MD: Aspen Publishers.

12. Turoff, M.P. (1949). *How to Make Pottery and Other Ceramic Ware*. New York: Crown Publishers.

13. Wilkinson, V.C. & Heater, S.L. (1979). *Therapeutic Media and Techniques of Application: A Guide for Activities Therapists*. New York: Van Nostrand Reinhold Company.

14. King, L.J. (1974). A sensory-integrative approach to schizophrenia. *American Journal of Occupational Therapy*, 28(9), 529-536.

15. Early, M.B. (1987). *Mental Health Concepts and Techniques for the Occupational Therapy Assistant*. New York: Raven Press.

16. Gaitskell, C.D. & Hurwitz, A. (1975). *Children and Their Art*, 3rd ed. New York: Harcourt, Brace, Jovanovitch.

17. Axline, V. (1947). *Play Therapy*. New York: Ballantine Books.

18. Weisberg, N. & Wilder, R. (1985). *Creative Arts With Older Adults: A Sourcebook*. New York: Human Sciences Press.

12
Weaving, Latchook, Macramé and Other Fiber Crafts

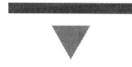

Introduction

Fiber crafts include much more than those mentioned in this chapter. To include all fiber crafts is out of the realm of this text. The most commonly used crafts for occupational therapy will be discussed with only two examples being described in detail.

Fiber Crafts Used in Occupational Therapy

Weaving

After leather, wood and ceramics, weaving may be the next craft that humans developed. It probably grew out of a tradition of basketry, which is also weaving. Grasses, reeds and leaves were probably the first woven fibers. Because of their vegetable nature, few of these early weaving artifacts have survived. The Middle Eastern cultures documented their crafts in artwork such as murals and commercial records such as clay tablets. We know that cloth was being woven in 4500 BC, however, almost all indigenous cultures have developed a form of weaving or basketry.[1-3]

Weaving can be as simple as paper weaving, which is dealt with in the next chapter, or it can be as complex as that done on a four-harness floor loom. Basically, no matter what the fiber, it is the same process—interweaving one set of strands with another set at right angles to it. The longitudinal threads are called the warp while the latitudinal strands are termed weft or woof.[4,5]

In the past, in occupational therapy clinics, it was common to see looms in use. There were often adapted looms to be used over a bed or positioned to require patients to use shoulder flexion, adduction and abduction.[1,6-8] It is possible for many looms to be "homemade."[2,9,10] Some kinds of weaving require little equipment, such as the inkle loom (Figure 12-1), finger weaving, card weaving and stick weaving. All of these are forms of strip weaving. The strips are then used as bracelets, belts, headbands and hat bands or are sewn together to make rugs or blankets. Knitting and crocheting are forms of making fabric without having threads interwoven at right angles. God's Eyes, which are a traditional Mexican and Indian decorative craft, are another kind of weaving that most beginners can do successfully.[11]

Latchook

Latchook is a modern adaptation of a common older style of rug-making called Turkish knotting or knotting, which can be made on any flat loom. It is a way of knotting fringe through two warp threads at a time. Row after row of fringe produces a nice pile rug.[1,2] Hooked rugs were often made with a burlap backing. A rug hook is a simple hook set in a wooden handle (Figure 12-2) and is used to pull loops of yarn up through the burlap to make a pile.[12]

Carpets today are essentially made in the same way though done by machine. Some have cut pile, which is like Turkish knotting and some have looped piles like hooked rugs.[1,5] A latchook is a special kind of hook with a small hinged appendage on it, which helps automatically knot the yarn as it is pulled through the rug canvas. The canvas is heavy

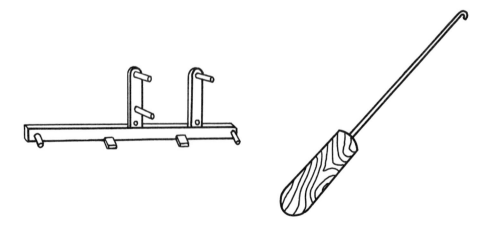

Figure 12-1
Inkle Loom

Figure 12-2
Rug Hook

woven white coarse cloth with large holes for inserting the latchook. It can be purchased in kits or rolls and cut to size. The yarn pieces used in latchooking are 2in. to 4in. in length. They can be purchased ready cut or they can be cut on a special yarn cutter that cuts the yarn directly from the skein. Latchook projects often take more time than is available in today's short stay hospital. However, once the process of latching is learned, it is an easy repetitive task. Latchook projects can be used for pillows, toilet covers, chair pads and rugs. Perhaps the most difficult part of latchooking is finishing the edges as the canvas is stiff and scratchy. Consequently it is difficult to fold over and stitch.

Macramé

This ancient craft of knotting was used by the pharonic Egyptians, the Chinese, the Maoris and the Peruvians. The word macramé has an Arabic origin meaning a veil of protection, a towel or napkin with a fringe. Because many of the knots used in macramé were also used by sailors, it is probable that the skill migrated to new places via the sea.[2,3]

Macramé can be accomplished with almost no tools. Some therapists use special macramé boards and pins, but this is not necessary. Many macramé projects are time consuming and consequently not appropriate for a short hospital stay. Simple projects can be done with tools already on hand in the clinic, such as scissors and masking tape.

In simple macramé there are four basic knots with several variations for each.[13] There are more than 30 complicated knots that can be incorporated if the activity needs to be graded up.[14] This craft can easily be graded up or down as the range of projects may include key chains, belts, purses, shopping bags, jewelry, wall hangings and plant pot hangers.[3]

Frequency of Use

Between 5% and 20% of therapists use macramé as often as one time per week or more. Many others use macramé occasionally or less than once a week.

In working on specific occupational therapy goals, weaving and latchook are often used to improve group socialization. Turkish knotting and knitting are used to increase bilateral dexterity. Latchook weaving and macramé are used to improve fine motor control. Some therapists use weaving to provide an outlet for frustration.

Assessments

Informal assessment of cognition, perceptual–motor, visual–perceptual and fine motor functions are possible using fiber crafts. Formal assessments usually do not use fibers. Perhaps this is because fiber crafts are an entirely new, complicated process to many patients. Such an evaluation, which would involve teaching the craft, would test only a narrow range of learning skills such as memory, following instructions, etc. The Neuropsychiatric Interest (NPI) Checklist includes knitting on its list of 80 activities. No other fiber arts except sewing and embroidery, which are classified in this text as needlework, are included. In the NPI Checklist the patient marks casual, strong or none to indicate the level of interest in each activity.[15]

Making Loopers

Loopers are simple squares woven of cotton or nylon jersey loops. Aside from paper weaving, they are the simplest weaving project. Perhaps that is why they are so commonly used.

Supplies
- Looper frame (Figure 12-3);
- Color assortment of loopers; and
- Wire looper hook.

PROCESS
Each side of the looper frame has 18 prongs.
1. Number each side of the frame.
2. Start on side one and slip a looper over the first prong and pull it across and hook it on the first prong directly across on side three.
3. Continue until loopers are hooked around the opposite prong on sides one and three. This is the warp.
4. To interweave the weft, starting on side two, slide the wire looper hook through the warp going under over, under over.
5. Slip the hook through the looper. Then slide the looper over the first prong on side two and pull the looper through the warp. Hook it on the side four prong opposite the one where it is hooked on side two.

Some consider each looper as one strand. It is perhaps less confusing for beginners to go under over under over, considering each side of one looper as a separate strand. Either way is satisfactory, though

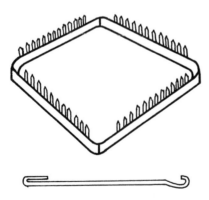

Figure 12-3
Looper Frame

the two-strand method gives a more vivid contrast of the colors. This plain weave is called ''tabby.'' Contrasting colors can be used to make a plaid effect. When each of the 18 weft loopers is woven through the warp and attached to the prongs at both sides, the square is ready to be removed.

6. Start at the same corner where the first warp looper was hooked over the prong on side one. Gently lift the next loop off the next prong.
7. Pull the second loop through the first. The hook will remain in the second loop ready to lift off the third loop and pull it through the second.
8. Continue until all loops are pulled through the previous loop. It may be necessary to pull a strand on the finished edge over a prong on each side to keep the square in place until the last loop is taken off the prong.
9. The finishing touch is to take another looper and put it through the last loop to make a hanger if the square is to be used as a potholder.
10. These squares can also be sewn together for rugs and placemats.[9]

Macramé Key Chain

Making macramé key chains is a simple project that can often be finished in one session to satisfy patients who need immediate gratification. The simplest key chain uses just two strands of cord. Macramé can be graded up from more strands on the key chain to complex wall hangings or clothing.

Supplies
- One split key ring;
- Two spools of different colored macramé cord;
- Assorted beads;
- Yardstick;
- Scissors; and
- Masking tape.

PROCESS
1. Tape the key ring to the table approximately 12in. from the edge at the place where the patient will sit.
2. Cut one yard of each color of cord.
3. Dip ends of cord in lacquer or nail polish so they won't fray during the macramé process. Allow these to dry. This is not always necessary but some patients tend to cause the cords to fray from too much handling. If the patient doesn't want

to put beads on the macramé, the ends can be separately knotted in overhand knots, to keep the ends from fraying.

4. Fold the cords in half and knot each strand through the key ring using a larkshead knot (Figure 12-4).
5. Tape the two center holding cords down to the table.
6. Lay the right-hand cord across the two holding cords and place the left under the holding cords; pull it over the right cord and through the loop (Figure 12-5).
7. Next lay the left cord across the two holding cords. Place the right end over the end of the left cord, under the holding cords and up through the loop (Figure 12-6).
8. Continue in this way.
9. After several knots, the patient may desire to put a bead on the two holding strands.
10. At this point, the two outer strands can be taped down and become the holding strands. Then the previous holding strands, which are longer at this point, are the ones used to make the knots as described above.
11. When the macramé reaches the desired length, cut off the extra cord.
12. The patient may want to put a bead near the end of each of the four strands and tie an overhand knot at the bottom to keep the beads from sliding off.

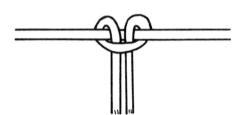

Figure 12-4
Larkshead Knot

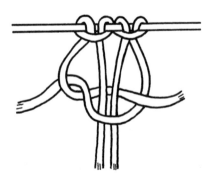

Figure 12-5
Square Knot Starting with the Right

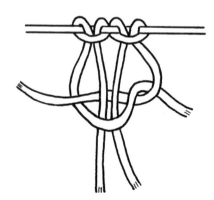

Figure 12-6
Square Knot Starting with the Left

Main Therapeutic Applications

Physical Dysfunction

Floor looms were once considered the most adaptable piece of craft equipment for working on range of motion, strength and endurance of both lower and upper extremities. They are seldom found in rehabilitation clinics now possibly because of the floor space requirements. Patients with ataxia or cerebellar dysfunction can practice movements in weaving that are normally controlled by the cerebellum such as starting, stopping and balance. Practice can allow the patient to learn to control these movements cortically. Those with hemiparesis can practice bilateral hand activity in all of the activities discussed in this chapter. The blind and deaf receive much tactile input through weaving and macramé. The small projects described in this chapter are easy to use in bed for confined patients. If patients have allergies or respiratory problems, caution needs to be used in choosing lint-free cord and yarn.

Mental Health

The simple fiber arts are appropriate for patients with poor attention spans. These activities are highly structured for patients who are, for example, schizophrenic and manic. These crafts offer quick gratification. They include simple skills that, once learned, can easily be built upon. Depressed patients who tire easily usually have enough endurance for these kinds of small projects. Latchook may seem a little more difficult to learn and certainly takes longer to complete. One precaution with fiber crafts is that suicidal patients many be tempted to try to hang themselves with cord. It is best not to let them take such projects to their rooms. The educable mentally retarded (IQ 50–70) who can achieve academic skills to the sixth grade can benefit from structured activities such as crochet, simple weaving, latchook and simple macramé. The repetitive nature of these crafts is nonthreatening to the retarded.[16]

Pediatrics

Fiber crafts are too difficult for most young children. Older children enjoy the simple fiber crafts. Boys may be motivated to try macramé as it will prepare them to learn nautical skills. Both boys and girls can enjoy weaving. If a boy suggests that it is not masculine, the therapist can describe how men do the weaving in countries like Saudi Arabia. Children may find latchook an especially satisfying activity if they work on the rug canvas with large holes using the very thickest yarn to make the pile plush enough. Simple patterns lend themselves to thick yarn.[17]

Geriatrics

Fiber activities are often chosen by older women. Many of them have had crotchet hooks or knitting needles in their hands since childhood. These activities, then, need little teaching. For older people, it is often best to let them do what they know well, as success in these activities can do much for failing self-esteem. Many men have learned to tie a variety of knots in their work or in home maintenance. This skill makes macramé a natural activity for them. They can craft gifts for friends or family.

Fiber crafts are inexpensive compared to wood, leather and ceramics. That makes such crafts attractive activities for use in nursing homes and other long-term-care facilities that have limited craft budgets.

Fiber crafts are not breakable. This is an important feature for geriatric patients who because of their balance problems, may drop things.[18]

Case Study

Helen is a 21-year-old white female who is classified as moderately mentally retarded with an IQ of 50. She lives with her parents in a suburban neighborhood. She is their only child remaining at home. For the past 12 years she has ridden a school bus for special education students across town to a school that has classes for the retarded. She also has epilepsy, which is controlled by medication.

For the past seven years, the school's occupational therapist has been working with Helen's teacher to develop her work skills in preparation for future placement in a sheltered workshop. At age 14, they started her on a program of standing for 15 minutes to do a repetitive task, gradually increasing her standing tolerance by five-minute increments. Some of the activities she did during this training were sorting colored objects, stringing beaded necklaces as gifts, making a link belt, using scissors to cut out coupons, and cooking simple dishes.

By the time she was 21 years old, she had a standing tolerance of two hours. At this age, she was no longer eligible for special education services so the occupational therapist worked with other school personnel to help Helen make a smooth transition to the sheltered workshop. She accompanied Helen on a visit to the workshop. The workshop had a full-time certified occupational therapy assistant (COTA) and a contract occupational therapist who spent four hours per week evaluating patients. The two occupational therapists set up a telephone conference about Helen. During her first two weeks at the workshop, she began to have seizures again. A call to her parents verified that she had been taking her medication. The workshop required that she start wearing her protective helmet again. Because her seizures had been controlled for so many years, she had not been made to wear it. The pediatrician whom Helen had been seeing for years consented to see her again, though he had been trying to get her referred to a family practice clinic that served many mentally retarded clients. The pediatrician began to alter her medication in an attempt to control the seizures.

The occupational therapist in the sheltered workshop evaluated Helen at the end of the second week and found her to be unkempt, sluggish and unresponsive. She got up and began to wander around the occupational therapy room during the evaluation. She started to go through the occupational therapist's desk saying "Candy Candy!" Her behavior did not fit with the description given by the school therapist. The workshop occupational therapist decided to call the school to discuss this situation. The outcome of this discussion was to try to reduce Helen's stress level by allowing her a more gradual integration into the workshop program. Usually, the workshop van brought the clients at 8:30 am. At 9:00 am, they started on the day's work. Each hour there was a ten minute break. At 11:00 am, the COTA taught a TMR vocational class. Helen was enrolled in this class. From 11:45 am to 12:30 pm, clients ate their lunch in the workshop cafeteria. At 12:30 pm they returned to work for two hours. From 2:30 until 3:30 pm, the COTA had a craft group for those clients who had been on time, dressed neatly and who had worked well.

The occupational therapist and COTA made the following goals and got Helen's agreement to work on these goals:

- To be punctual at her work station;
- To be neatly dressed and groomed;
- To stay at her work station for 50 minutes; and
- To finish one task before starting another.

It was decided that the COTA could work on some of these skills in the TMR vocational class and she could decide on Helen's rewards in the craft session. Helen had initially indicated interest in several crafts. She had never done looper weaving. At the next session, the COTA had Helen sort out loopers for weaving into four separate colors and put each color in a separate bag. The next day she allowed Helen to choose the two colors she would like to use in her own looper. She chose a blue and green. Though the COTA felt they did not look good together, she did not interfere because she felt Helen needed more independent decision making. At that session Helen put the blue warp loopers on the loom. The following day, Helen completed weaving the green weft loopers. On the third day, she had difficulty with the process of removing the loops from the prongs and hooking them through the previous loop. The COTA had to sit beside her to see that she was doing it correctly. Finally, after she reached the fourth side of the loom, she seemed to catch on to this process. She was proud of the completed potholder and took it to show each person in the clinic saying "Isn't it pretty?" She told the COTA she wanted to make another one. The COTA said if she came to her work station on time and was neat and clean she could start another the next day. Helen responded positively to this agreement. Her seizures began to diminish and eventually disappeared. It was felt by all the workshop staff that the simple repetitive nature of looper weaving seemed to calm Helen and reduced her stress, which was believed to have set off the seizures. While Helen did later learn other crafts, nothing seemed to please her like loopers.

Discussion Questions

1. What particular features of loopers might appeal so strongly to Helen?
2. How could the COTA grade up loopers to keep a higher-functioning patient interested and challenged?
3. Which of the fiber crafts described in this chapter requires the greatest range of motion?

References

1. Department of the Army. (1971). *Craft Techniques in Occupational Therapy.* Washington DC: US Government Printing Office.
2. Moseley, S., Johnson, P., & Koenig, H. (1962). *Crafts Design.* Belmont, CA: Wadsworth.
3. Reader's Digest. (1979). *Crafts and Hobbies.* Pleasantville, NY: The Reader's Digest Association Inc.
4. Hedrick, S.J. (Ed.). (1971). *What Shall I Weave?* Shelby, NC: Lily Mills Company.
5. Scharff, R. (1952). *Handbook of Crafts.* Greenville, CT: Fawcett Publications.
6. Colson, J.H.C. (1944). *The Rehabilitation of the Injured: Occupational Therapy.* London: Cassell and Company.
7. Haworth, N.A. & Macdonald, E.M. (1946). *Theory of Occupational Therapy.* Baltimore: Williams & Wilkins.
8. Willard, H.S. & Spackman, C.E. (1947). *Principles of Occupational Therapy.* Philadelphia: Lippincott.
9. Alexander, M. (1969). *Simple Weaving.* New York: Tower Publications.
10. Harding, D. (February, 1973). Weaving with a simple stick loom. *Family Circle,* 81: 152, 154.
11. Stribling, M.L. (1973). *Art From Found Materials.* New York: Crown Publishers, Inc.
12. Better Homes and Gardens. (1966). *Stitchery and Crafts.* New York: Meredith Press.
13. Octopus Books. (1973). *The Basic Book of Macramé and Tatting.* Hong Kong: Mandarin Publishers.
14. Abraham, R.M. (1964). *Diversions and Pastimes with Coins, Cards, String, Paper and Matches.* New York: Dover Publications.
15. Matsutsuya, J.S. (1969). The interest checklist. *American Journal of Occupational Therapy,* 24(4).
16. American Psychiatric Association. (1987). *Diagnostic and Statistical Manual of Mental Disorders,* 3rd ed., revised. Washington DC: American Psychiatric Association: Author.
17. MacFarlan, A.S. (1973). *The Boys' Book of Rainy-Day-Doings.* New York: Galahad Books.
18. Gould, E. & Gould, L. (1971). *Crafts for the Elderly.* Springfield, IL: Charles C. Thomas Publisher.

Part

III

*Nontraditional Crafts
and Minor Media
Activities Used
Clinically in Therapy*

▼

13
Paper Crafts

Introduction

Paper was invented in China sometime between 200 and 100 BC. Other materials had been used to write on for many centuries before that: wet clay, tree bark, cloth, and papyrus, from which the word paper comes. Early paper was used almost solely to write on. The Arabs who learned about paper from their conquests in Asia, introduced it to Europe.

Paper was still being made by hand at the time of the invention of the printing press in the 15th century. In the 18th century, a machine was invented that could make paper from wood pulp though it did not become widely used for another 100 years. During these same centuries, the Chinese had been developing glue that they used to fashion many paper crafts. The Chinese continue to make cut paper ornaments from recycled paper even today. The Japanese craft of paper folding, origami, became increasingly sophisticated and today there is the tradition of groups joining in folding 1,000 paper cranes as expressions of peace and love. Mexican paper cutouts are intricate and colorful. The French developed the craft of paper maché or *chewed paper*.

Paper is perhaps our cheapest and most available craft material. Almost every office has a supply of paper, pencil, glue, scissors, tape and staples and paper clips, all that are needed for many projects. Most of us have been doing paper crafts for so long, we seldom think of them as important but they can be adapted for almost any patient population. Our parents may have kept us quiet at church, mosque or temple by folding paper boats. We learned how to outwit our teachers by flying paper airplanes. Our earliest party and holiday decorations may have been paper chains. Paper, aside from its important function for writing, offers a world of craft delight for all ages.[1-3]

Frequency of Use

Collage, decoupage and nature printing are among the most commonly used paper crafts. Only one of these, collage, will be discussed in this chapter. The paper crafts described here are mostly three-dimensional crafts or at least those involving folding the paper before cutting it. While folded paper crafts may be less commonly used than other crafts such as woodworking, they have the remarkable potential to increase eye-hand coordination, spatial relations, fine motor control, sequencing and other cognitive processes such as memory. The low cost of this treatment material is another reason for therapists to use it more frequently.

Assessments

Perhaps because paper crafts do not seem sophisticated to therapists, or therapists think patients may consider such activities as beneath them in relation to their age, few formal assessments include paper crafts. The Fidler Activity Laboratory[4] includes two paper activities. The first is a drawing of a chicken, which the client is asked to cut out and reproduce on another sheet of paper. The second is a collage using a variety of colored paper, objects and glue. The first offers almost no opportunity for creativity but the second activity can be quite imaginative. Other activities in this battery include fingerpainting and negotiating an obstacle course.

The Build-a-City assessment is a projective test meant primarily for testing a group of children. The assessment's author, however, lists the age span for the assessment from adolescent to geriatric. This assessment does work especially well with children. Colored construction paper along with tape, string, clay, pipe cleaners, scissors and clay tools are provided. The therapists simply asks the group of five to eight clients to build an ideal city. Interaction, fine motor function and approach to the task can be assessed.[5]

The Lafayette Clinic Battery[6] for children six to ten years of age uses construction paper, scissors, pencils, paste and circle patterns to test eye-hand coordination. The test also includes a geometric form worksheet and puzzle. This assessment evaluates the child's developmental skills.

The Magazine Picture Collage is an adult psychiatric occupational therapy evaluation. In this assessment, the patient is given colored construction paper, a pile of magazines, scissors and glue. The patient is asked to look for pictures that appeal to him or her and to glue them to the construction paper. This assessment has been well-validated for interrater reliability.[4]

Paper Maché

Paper maché can be made by several different processes: by soaking pieces of torn up newspaper and mixing it with cooked starch; by using commercially prepared paper maché mix or by using the strip method. The last method will be discussed here, as illustrated by the creation of a paper maché wall mask.

Supplies
- Paper plate;
- Newspapers;
- Masking tape;
- Liquid white glue;
- Bowl to mix glue; and
- Tempra paints and brushes.

PROCESS
1. Cover the work space with several thicknesses of newspaper.
2. Make a mask form by loosely wadding several pieces of newspaper and taping them into the top of the paper plate to make the general shape of a face.
3. If a nose or other appendage such as ears or beard are desired, small wads of paper can be taped on the form.
4. Cover as much of the surface with tape as possible as it will allow the finished mask to be more easily removed from the plate and the wadded paper.
5. Tear up one sheet of black and white newspaper into strips approximately 1in. wide.
6. In the bowl, mix one part white glue to one part water.
7. Dip each strip in the glue and apply it to the mask form. Allow this to dry thoroughly before applying the next layer of strips. This may take 24 hours.
8. For the next layer, tear strips from the colored comics strip section so that when the glued strips are applied, it is easy to see that all the surface has been covered with the second layer. Allow this to dry also. The third and last layer of strips should be of plain black and white newspaper.
9. After the third layer is dry, smooth the mask by sanding the surface lightly or by adding additional strips to rough spots.
10. Pull off the paper plate and wadded paper when the mask is completely dry.
11. Paint the mask with any water-based paint.
12. Lacquer the mask to keep the paint from wearing off.

If the mask is to be worn, rather than hung on the wall, leave eye holes on the very first and subsequent layers. It is better not to try to cut the completely dried mask as it may crack.[2,3]

Paper Weaving

This craft is appropriate for almost any age. It can help assess and improve patients' awareness of space, awareness of under and over, fine motor coordination and motor planning. The process for making a simple woven placemat is described below.

Supplies
- Two- 12in. by 18in. sheets of different colored construction paper;
- Scissors (be sure to have left-handed scissors available); and
- White glue.

PROCESS
1. Decide on which color the background or warp will be as described in the chapter on fiber crafts.
2. Fold that sheet lengthwise down the middle.
3. Mark the edge opposite the fold so there is a 1/2in. margin.
4. Start from the fold and cut to the margin, making cuts 3/4in. apart (Figure 13-1).
5. Open up the sheet and lay it flat.
6. From the other sheet cut 3/4in. lengthwise weft strips (Figure 13-2).
7. To make a plain tabby weave, just take one weft strip and go under over, under over.
8. The next strip will be over under, over under.
9. Continue weaving, alternating these patterns until there is no more room for a weft to be woven into the warp (Figure 13-3).
10. Lightly glue the ends of each weft strip.

Folded Paper

The Japanese are famous for their origami figures. Because it is a traditional craft in Japan, almost every Japanese school child learns to do some figures. Animals, flowers, puppets, boxes and abstract forms are all subjects for the origami crafter. Many of these forms can be adapted for use in the clinic. The cat shown in the illustrations below is one of the simplest figures. It is possible to buy special origami paper but any thin paper such as typing paper can be used.

PROCESS
1. Fold an 8in. square of paper from corner to corner (Figure 13-4).
2. Next fold the top corner so the crease comes 2in. from the top corner (Figures 13-5 and 13-6).

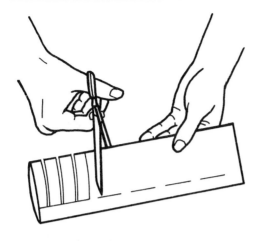

Figure 13-1
Cutting Warp for Paper Weaving

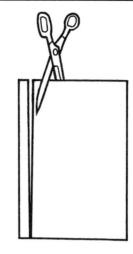

Figure 13-2
Cutting Weft for Paper Weaving

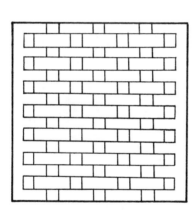

Figure 13-3
Completed Paper Weaving

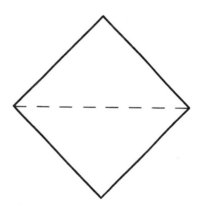

Figure 13-4
Origami Cat, First Fold

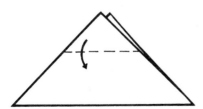

Figure 13-5
Origami Cat, Second Fold

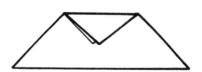

Figure 13-6
Origami Cat, Second Fold Completed

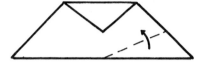

Figure 13-7
Origami Cat, Third Fold

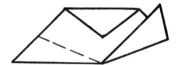

Figure 13-8
Origami Cat, Fourth and Final Fold

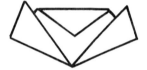

Figure 13-9
Back of Origami Cat Face

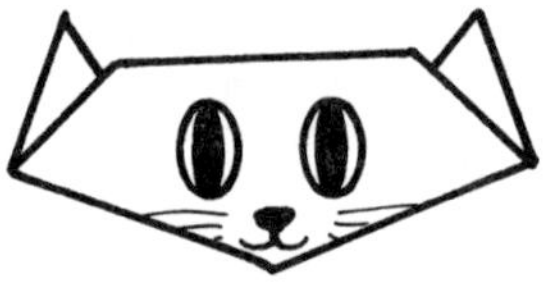

Figure 13-10
Front of Origami Cat Face Drawn
on with Felt Pen

3. Fold the ears up (Figures 13-7 and 13-8 and 13-9) and turn the cat's head over.
4. Draw eyes, nose, mouth and whiskers. The cat's face can be decorated in a number of different ways (Figure 13-10).[7]

Paper Sculpture

Paper sculpture offers an infinite variety for stimulating creativity. Subjects can be realistic, futuristic, imaginative or abstract. Glue is the next most important material after paper for this kind of sculpture.[8,9] Sculpture implies that it is a three-dimensional object. Sculpture can be constructed from a pattern (Figure 13-11) or it can be built by adding paper to an understructure. The piñata described below uses the latter technique. A piñata is a Mexican holiday sculpture used in a game. The outcome of the game is a broken piñata but it can be appropriate fun in some situations.

Supplies
- Two large brown paper bags;
- Cellophane tape;
- Large needles and string;
- Assorted wrapped candies;
- Colored tissue paper;
- Glue;
- Water; and
- Scissors.

PROCESS
1. Fit one paper bag inside the other.
2. Fold 2in. of the tops of both bags down inside the bags.
3. Place a strip of cellophane tape on the middle where the string will go through. That will reinforce the paper so the string won't tear the bags as easily.
4. Now, accordion fold the folded top of the bags (Figure 13-12).
5. Put needle and string through this taped strip.
6. Fill the double bag with candy to approximately 5in. from the top.
7. Pull the string to close the top of the bag. Leave the extra string at the top to hang it by. Now the piñata structure is ready to be covered with fringed paper. This shape makes a

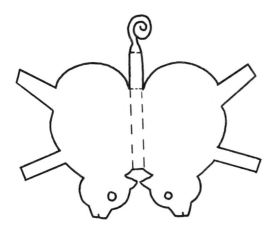

Figure 13-11
Paper Sculpture Pattern

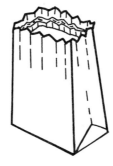

Figure 13-12
Accordion-Folded Bag with
Taped Strip for Piñata

nice piece of fruit like an apple or a berry.

8. The piñata can be hung up during the gluing process. Take a 4in. by 24in. length of tissue paper and fold it down the middle.

9. Cut 1/4in. widths (Figure 13-13) the length of the strip.

10. Glue the uncut edges of the folded paper to the piñata structure starting at the bottom and working in a spiral until the whole piñata is covered. Use the glue sparingly, spreading it with a small brush.

11. Near the string add a few rows of green fringe to make it look like a fruit stem. Allow the piñata to dry for at least 24 hours.

The piñata game is played by tying a rope to the piñata string so it can be pulled up or let down lower. A basketball hoop makes a good place to hang a piñata so there is enough space underneath to play the game. All the players form a big circle around the piñata. Each player is blindfolded in turn. They are led to the center of the circle and given one-half or one-fourth of a turn before they are allowed to try to break the piñata (Figure 13-14). Care must be taken that all the players in the circle stay far out of the reach of the stick. Turns are taken hitting at the piñata until someone breaks it and the candy falls on the ground. All players share the candy. This Mexican game is often played at Christmas. It can also be played at any special occasion such as a patient's birthday.

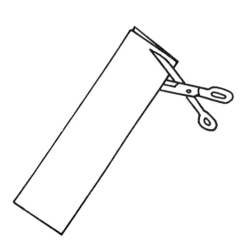

Figure 13-13
Cutting the Folded Edge of the Tissue Paper Strip

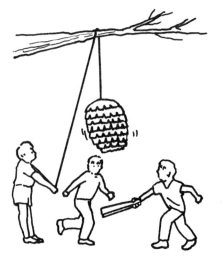

Figure 13-14
Children Breaking the Piñata

Main Therapeutic Applications

Physical Dysfunction

Paper crafts can be structured for almost any health care situation. They are especially appropriate for home health patients as the materials are usually available and not costly to replace. Most of the paper crafts emphasize finger, wrist, forearm and elbow movement. While little strength is required in most cases, endurance may be required to hold pieces of paper in a position until the glue or starch sticks. Paper crafts are especially good for cardiac and respiratory patients as little exertion is required. All motion can be done in the lap. The materials give off no toxic fumes. Almost all paper crafts require bilateral hand function.

Mental Health

Paper craft is potentially frustrating as paper can tear or be crushed readily. The therapist must be very alert to those patients who need closer supervision to prevent failure. Psychiatric patients often have difficulty judging how much glue to use. Applying the glue with a small brush may help with this problem.

Simple paper folding can be used to assess cognitive function, ability to follow directions, spacial awareness and frustration tolerance. For the higher-functioning patient, paper sculpture can be used as a projective test in the same way that other sculpture is used. The patients can be asked to describe their sculpture and indicate what meaning it has for them.

Paper crafts make wonderful holiday decorations. Hanging ornaments, flowers, garlands, streamers and mobiles all help to bring a holiday mood to a clinic or dayroom. Most paper crafts, except paper weaving and paper chains, will be too difficult for mentally retarded clients. However, they may enjoy drawing around stencils, cutting them out and pasting them onto another color of paper.

Pediatrics

Paper crafts are especially good for children as they can use their own creations as toys. Very young children can tear paper but they very quickly want to use scissors. They can make paper puppets or paper bag puppets who do their talking for them, which is especially appropriate for children having difficulty communicating. They can build a world, destroy it and rebuild it as they do in their fantasies. They can make their own family members or pets and do to them whatever they fantasize as an emotional release.

One of the greatest problems for children is that they use too much glue. Paste may be better for young children though it does not hold as well. Cone-based structures are best for paper sculpture as there usually are no balance problems. Children are particularly likely to form sculptures with a base too small to support them. Children often want to embellish their paper craft with paint or crayon. Encouragement of such creativity will foster more exploration of materials and possibilities. As children approach adolescence they want to make more realistic sculptures. Paper craft does not lend itself to realism in most situations. Drawing may be better for this age. However, teens can excel at mask making, origami and sculpture.[10]

Geriatrics

Paper and fabric can often be used to make similar designs. Quilt patterns and appliqués that may have been used by the patients in the past can easily be adapted to paper designs. Few older patients like to experiment, so the kinds of projects they will enjoy are often fairly familiarly structured activities. Even the most disabled patients in nursing homes often enjoy pasting precut flowers into a bouquet or precut holly leaves into a wreath. This offers opportunities for ensured success. Making paper toys for children may provide stimulation for some elderly patients. Paper crafts may be difficult for a patient with vision problems. Folding paper could stress severely deformed arthritic finger and hand joints. Paper cuts on the edge of the paper are painful and annoying. Particular precautions need to be take with the elderly patients who heal more slowly.

Case Study

In a children's mental health unit with a bed capacity of ten, the occupational therapist did almost all patient evaluation and treatment in a group setting. Most of the patients had the diagnosis of conduct disorder though occasionally there were others. The program had strict behavioral limits. Children earned privileges such as television or playground time through accomplishing goals for each treatment session, mealtime and therapeutic community meeting.

There was an adolescent treatment unit next door. Patients were placed in whichever program they best fit behaviorally. The average length of stay was three weeks. The occupational therapist split her time between these two psychiatric units. On the children's unit, she customarily evaluated each child individually on the Meeting Street School Screening Test[11] to assess information processing capabilities and gross and fine motor development. The Draw-A-Person test was administered in a group if possible as was the Build-a-City assessment.

Since programming was slightly less structured on weekends and children were often discharged before weekends, the evaluation was usually done by Friday to ensure enough children for a group. A certified occupational therapy assistant (COTA) came in for four hours each weekend day to do the occupational therapy treatment programs.

Seven-year-old Ronald was admitted on a Friday, which was an unusual occurrence. The hospital usually tried not to make admissions on Friday so new patients would not come into the less-structured weekend program. However, Ronald's single mother said she could not care for him another minute. She had three younger children living with her in her mother's house. Her mother is unable to help her with child care as she is physically disabled. Ronald had been attacking his younger siblings and endangering himself by jumping off high places and riding his bike off cement culverts. He was just recovering from a broken arm. The psychiatrist diagnosed Ronald as suffering from depression with conduct disorder.

The occupational therapist administered the Meeting Street School Screening Test and found Ronald performed normally on gross and fine motor tasks though his responses were sometimes slightly delayed. There was some interference in his information processing. Though he performed tasks adequately he seemed inattentive. His projective story about the two figures involved stealing a cat and hurting it.

The therapist had to postpone the other two tests. She discussed Ronald's condition by telephone with the weekend COTA. On Monday morning, Tom and Paul, two brothers aged six and eight years, were admitted. They had been taken from their foster home and brought to the hospital by the case worker. They had both been seen before by the psychiatrist in the psychiatric daycare but this was their first hospital admission. They were both diagnosed as conduct disorders.

Their mother had abandoned them and their father felt unable to care for them. He came to visit them in foster placement but avoided answering them when they asked him when they could go with him. His visit on Saturday had precipitated the current crisis in the foster home. They had been fighting and abusing the five-year-old daughter of the foster mother.

The occupational therapist decided to conduct her two group assessments at her first session. She started the Draw-A-Person test by placing the boys as far from each other as possible at the primary-sized table. They all drew hurriedly. The two brothers made frequent aggressive comments to each other. While an aide took the boys for a snack, the therapist assembled the materials for the Build-a-City assessment. She had empty thread spools, plasticene modeling clay, tape, glue, construction paper, colored pencils, string, scissors, blunt table knives, wooden clay modeling tools and styrofoam cubes. She gave them the direction to build an ideal city in 45 minutes. The boys all began to grab items from the table. They worked individually for some minutes. Ronald began to draw and cut out cars. Paul began to draw a house. Tom dropped his own attempt at taping sheets of construction paper together for a street map and grabbed Paul's picture saying "Let me show you how to make a house." He turned Paul's paper over and folded the sides of the paper to make a three-dimensional rectangle. Then he taped the folds in place and threw it back to Paul saying "Cut a door and some windows, stupid!" The therapist was tempted to intervene but decided to wait until after the evaluation was over. The hostile interaction between the two brothers soon included Ronald as well. Tom had taken charge and the other two boy chafed under his dictatorial manner but neither resisted him physically. The completed city was three sheets of gray construction paper taped together. Strips of black paper were glued on top of the gray paper as streets. There were four blue and yellow rectangular paper houses and a red McDonald Hamburger shop. Tom had made three clay human figures that he stood up between the houses. Ronald's six cars and two trucks were two dimensional and were propped up on the streets between small balls of clay.

In the discussion following their work, the boys frequently interrupted each other as they tried to explain the importance of each object. Tom invariably won out and explained for the other boys. Ronald was able to demonstrate two cars crashing at a corner and in the process squashed one of Tom's clay people. Tom began to hit Ronald but the therapist intervened and helped them clean up paper scraps. Each boy earned a checkmark for cleaning up. She sent the boys to the dayroom with an aide. Tom and Paul were each assessed individually with the Meeting Street Test. Impulsiveness was their greatest problem.

In the afternoon session, she decided to help the boys make two paper bag puppets each so they could begin to act out their anger and aggression in a structured way. The boys drew eyes, noses, mouths and other features with felt pens. They pasted paper, yarn and pieces of cloth for hats and clothes. The next day, each boy was invited to give a puppet show with his two paper bag puppets. By the third puppet show, Tom asked Ronald to help him by handling and being one of his puppets. This was a positive sign of learning to cooperate. The boys were rewarded with checkmarks for improved cooperation. The therapist felt that paper crafts might be used often with the boys during the next week along with a variety of other activities.

Discussion Questions

1. What reason would the therapist have for not intervening when the boys verbally abused each other during the Build-a-City assessment?
2. Had the therapist chosen to start the boys out at the second session making paper maché masks instead of puppets, what kind of problems do you think she might have encountered?
3. It is common for children to make gifts for their parents. What might you suggest to these three boys to make for their parents?

References

1. Department of the Army. (1971). *Craft Techniques in Occupational Therapy.* Washington DC: US Government Printing Office.
2. Moseley, S., Johnson, P., & Koenig, H. (1962). *Crafts Design.* Belmont, CA: Wadsworth.
3. Reader's Digest. (1979). *Crafts and Hobbies.* Pleasantville, NY: The Reader's Digest Association Inc.
4. Hemphill, B.J. (1982). The Evaluative Process in Psychiatric Occupational Therapy. Thorofare, NJ: Slack.
5. Practice Division. (1988). *Mental Health Information Packet.* Rockville, MD: American Occupational Therapy Association.
6. Llorens, L.A. (1969). An evaluation procedure for children 6-10 years of age. *American Journal of Occupational Therapy,* 21(2), 64-69.
7. Sakade, F. (1958). *Origami: Book Two: Japanese Paper-Folding.* Rutland, VT: Charles E. Tuttle Company.
8. Bottomley, J. (1983). *Paper Projects for Creative Kids of All Ages.* Boston: Little, Brown and Company.
9. Fabri, R. (1966). *Sculpture in Paper.* New York: Watson-Guptill Publications.
10. Gaitskell, C.D. & Hurwitz, A. (1975). *Children and Their Art,* 3rd ed. New York: Harcourt, Brace, Jovanovitch.
11. Hainsworth, P.K. & Siqueland, M.L. (1969). *Early Identification of Children With Learning Disabilities: The Meeting Street School Screening Test.* East Providence, RI: The Easter Seal Society for Crippled Children and Adults of Rhode Island.

14
Cooking as a Craft

Introduction

The first sentence of this book defines craft as "an occupation requiring special skill" and a skill as "a learned power of doing a thing competently."[1] These descriptions obviously put cooking into the craft category. Food, after air and water, is our greatest need. This is undoubtedly one of the reasons there are more cookbooks published than any other category of text and why cooking is the most commonly practiced craft in all occupational therapy clinics. Everyone has to eat.

How did cooking start? Many of us have undoubtedly been raised with Charles Lamb's story about the first roast pig in which the man's house burned and cooked the pig's flesh, which the man then tasted. More probably the homo erectus were the first primates to cook. Cooking makes foods tasty, less tough, and allows them to keep longer. Perhaps these reasons motivated homo erectus to expand on this craft. First attempts probably were similar to Charles Lamb's tale. Homo erectus may have simply laid a joint of meat on the coals of a fire by mistake, then ran to recover it, tasted it and said "yum yum."

Neanderthals apparently developed stews by hanging a skin of water and meat over a fire. The wet leather would not burn but the heat would boil the stew. Neolithic humans evidently developed the technique of dropping hot stones into a pit of water to cook grains. The development of ceramic pots helped in the refinement of early cooking. Discovery of the properties of metal would have carried the development of food preparation to an even more skilled level as would ovens and fireplaces in which heat could be more controlled than it could in an open fire. This process of improved efficiency continued with development of food preservation, cooking stoves, refrigerators and on up into the era of microwaves.[2,3]

Our own cultural background greatly affects what foods we choose. Cultural foods are affected by economics, climate and growing season, geological aspects of soil and water, and food ideas our ancestors brought with them from their previous homes.[4] Often when we crave something in particular, it relates back to early food experiences. For example, to some people peanut butter and graham crackers bring back feelings of childhood mid-morning snack time.

Many people attribute eating problems to early associations with food. Food a person once enjoyed may come to seem like a necessity. They unconsciously desire the former good feeling associated with eating that food and want to achieve it again by repeating the food experience expecting to get the same emotional experience.[5,6] A way to think about food and cooking is to use Maslow's Hierarchy of Human Needs (Figure 6-1), illustrated in Chapter 6. Food can be used in an attempt to fulfill the needs expressed at any level. At the lowest level, food and cooking can be for nutrition. At the level of love and belonging, many people associate cooking with a mother's care and family dinners.

Success and self-esteem on the next level can be expressed by eating in nice restaurants. On the highest level, self-actualization is expressed by many men and women by doing creative cooking. An activity associated with food can appeal to a patient functioning at almost any level. Food and cooking can be used to accomplish occupational therapy goals with almost all patients.

Frequency of Use

Cooking is used by seven out of ten therapists in clinics. This craft is used more than any other. It is used to improve bilateral dexterity and to encourage self-expression. Mealtimes, eating and homemaking are also used to increase socialization and improve fine motor control. Nonetheless, cooking traditionally was seldom mentioned in occupational therapy literature.[7-11] This important craft, which is used more than any other, has had little formal acknowledgment.

Assessments

Cooking evaluations have been included as part of occupational therapy homemaking assessments for some time.[12-15] These evaluations assess capability to perform the physical and mental processes involved in food preparation. A wide variety of homemaker checklists exist. A cooking evaluation was often seen as part of career rehabilitation assessment for the homemaker. Commonly, a woman was asked to prepare a cake mix, a tuna salad or a simple casserole. As men's and women's roles have expanded, evaluating cooking skills has become an important consideration for all adults not living in institutions with communal dining. Perhaps the role changes for both men and women are an underlying cause for cooking being the most used craft activity.

Current evaluations that include cooking as a part of assessment are The Jacobs Prevocational Skills Assessment, The Scoreable Self-Care Evaluation, Instrumental Activities of Daily Living Scale, Comprehensive Evaluation of Basic Living Skills, The Interest Checklist, and The Street Survival Skills Questionnaire. Food preparation is the last of 15 tasks in the Jacobs Prevocational Skills Assessment. Patients are presented with materials and illustrated instructions for making honey butter and crackers. They are timed and scored on 15 performance areas. They do get to eat the crackers at the end.[16]

Actual cooking performance is not done in the Scoreable Self-Care Evaluation but there is a *foods selection* section. It involves choosing and planning menus for all meals for two days. The patient is scored on whether the menus are nutritionally balanced. For kitchen clean-up, the patient is asked to place ten task cards in sequence.

In The Instrumental Activities of Daily Living Scale (IADL), food preparation is one of eight tasks scored for degree of independence. It is an assessment for older adults. The therapist observes the patient doing the various tasks and rates performance on a dependence/independence scale.[17,18]

On The Comprehensive Evaluation of Basic Living Skills, the client is observed while doing meal planning, shopping, meal preparation, serving, eating and clean-up as well as using the telephone and taking a public bus. Each component of each task is rated from unable to perform to independently and correctly.[17]

The Neuropsychiatric Institute (NPI) Interest Checklist includes barbecues and cooking on its list of 80 activities that patients rate for their interest level. In the discussion following the completion of the list, this can be a stimulator for discussion of leisure choices. Such checklists are used in one in four of all psychiatric occupational therapy departments.[19] A positive response on the Interest Checklist about cooking will offer an opportunity to persuade a patient to participate in a cooking activity in the occupational therapy kitchen.

The Street Survival Skills Questionnaire is a test of adaptive skills in nine basic areas. Domestics is the area that includes 12 questions on cooking. The patient is shown pictures and asked questions about food preparation processes related to the pictures. There is a curriculum guide that has lessons to use to teach the areas for which deficits are found.[20]

Food Projects

The projects presented here are graded from simple to more complex. These recipes could hopefully be eaten by most hospitalized patients. If there is any doubt about whether a specific patient can eat a particular food, consult the patient's physician.

Simple Food Project: Stuffed Celery

Supplies
- Washed and trimmed 4in. stalks of celery;
- Nonhydrogenated peanut butter;
- Softened cream cheese; and
- Metal table knife.

Since this is a simple one-step process: the therapist will need to have previously washed, trimmed and cut the celery to 4in. lengths. The only step for a patient is to evenly spread the peanut butter or cheese into the groove in the celery. A second step could be to attractively arrange the stuffed celery on a plate. Food projects as simple as this could be used with young children, with the trainable mentally retarded or for anyone working on bilateral fine motor activities.

Easy Food Project: Pasta Salad

Supplies
- 8oz. package of pasta;
- 2 cups of cubed cooked meat, such as chicken;
- 1 cup of sliced raw vegetables, such as broccoli, celery, carrots or tomatoes; and
- 1 cup of salad dressing.

Equipment
- Stove and refrigerator;
- 2qt. pot with lid;
- 2 1-cup measuring cups;
- 2 sharp cutting knives;
- 2 cutting boards;
- Drainer;
- Large salad bowl; and
- Serving spoon.

PROCESS
1. Cook the pasta according to the directions on the package.
2. Drain, rinse and allow pasta to drain again in the drainer.
3. Mix the pasta, meat and vegetables in a large bowl.
4. Pour the dressing over and stir gently.
5. Chill in refrigerator. This recipe makes six servings.[21]

This recipe might be used as a group cooking project in which one patient cooks and rinses the pasta, another cubes the meat, another slices the vegetables and a fourth mixes the ingredients. It could be served as part of a meal cooked by a group as part of a nutrition or socialization session. Because the process involves potentially danger-ous activities—boiling food and cutting with sharp knives—patients need close supervision. If the session is one on a psychiatric unit, a tool count needs to be completed after dishes are washed and before any patients leave in order to prevent self-injurious incidents.

More Complex Project: Salt-Free Wheat Bread
This bread recipe has no salt, very little sweetening and almost no cholesterol.

Ingredients
- 1 package of dry yeast;
- 1/4 cup of lukewarm water;
- 1 1/4 cups all-purpose flour;
- 1 1/4 cups wholewheat flour;
- 2 tablespoons of molasses;
- 3/4 cup of lukewarm skim milk;
- 2 tablespoons of vegetable oil; and
- 2 teaspoons margarine.

PROCESS
1. Grease the loaf pan with one teaspoon of the margarine using fingers; wash margarine off hands. Nonstick cooking spray may be substituted for margarine.
2. Test lukewarm water by dropping a drop on the inner wrist to determine if it is at body temperature, which is lukewarm. Stir in the molasses. Sprinkle the yeast over this mixture and stir until it is dissolved. Allow it to stand.
3. Measure the two kinds of flour into a bowl.
4. Mix the flour evenly and make a crater in the middle.
5. Pour the yeast mixture, the lukewarm milk and the oil into the crater and mix until the dough is smooth.
6. Turn the dough out onto a counter top that has a thin layer of flour on it.
7. Knead the dough by quickly pressing to flatten it slightly, then folding it over and flattening and folding. Continue this process for two minutes. Keep the counter top lightly dusted with flour.
8. Form a ball with the dough.
9. With the other teaspoon of margerine, grease a mixing bowl, or spray it with nonstick cooking spray.
10. Place the dough in the bowl and turn it over to coat it with margerine. Lay a cloth or paper towel over the bowl to protect the dough from drafts of cold air as well as from dust.
11. Put the bowl in a warm place to allow the dough to rise for 1 hour.
12. Put the dough back on the floured counter and punch it down.
13. Form a loaf shape and place it in the greased pan. Cover it and allow the dough to rise for 45 minutes.

14. Preheat oven to 350°F.
15. Bake the loaf 30 minutes.
16. Remove the pan from the oven and place it on a wire rack to cool for ten minutes.
17. Turn the pan over to get the bread out.

For patients on restricted diets, learning to make their own bread can be very helpful. To perform this activity adequately, the patient would need at least three hours, enough sensory reception to be able to determine temperature, to be able to follow written or oral directions and to be able to keep the tasks in sequence, to be able to read numbers, and to be able to remember time limits for waiting and baking. A kitchen timer many be helpful for this aspect of the activity. It is possible to bake this loaf in a toaster oven if a 7in. by 11in. rectangular pan is used. If the occupational therapy clinic does not have a kitchen, a toaster oven, or microwave oven can offer many cooking possibilities.

Main Therapeutic Applications

Physical Dysfunction

For the sick person unable to do many things, food often becomes a focus of much attention. If the disability causes a disturbance in the eating process itself, for example, in a stroke, spinal cord injury, or head and neck surgery, helping the patient with choosing appropriate foods is an important activity.

Weight control or diabetic diets may be important issues to deal with in using cooking as treatment with patients. Planning meals and practicing cooking can be major activities patients need to do to prove to themselves that they will be able to surmount their problem and continue to enjoy life.[22] With neurological patients, cooking can be useful in dealing with safety issues, mobility, balance and cognitive deficits such as memory, judgment and sequencing. For the blind, managing in the kitchen where there are so many possible hazards is a primary area of treatment concern. There are many aids and adaptive devices for patients who need this kind of help with food preparation. Companies who sell adaptive equipment of this kind are listed in Appendix I.

Mental Health

Because food is so often tied to our early experiences of feeling loved and nurtured, cooking provides a rich opportunity to patients to relearn to nurture themselves. Depressed patients often have little appetite and may be difficult to coax to participate. Sometimes the involvement of a whole group in cooking will draw them in. Special care must be observed with suicidal patients when they are using sharp tools. Manic patients often want to cook elaborate dishes or meals. They may become distracted before they have progressed far with their task.

Schizophrenics may be slow about doing the cooking task they are assigned. They will need close supervision as with all mental health patients. For those who have eating disorders such as anorexia nervosa, bulimia or obesity, a cooking activity is an opportunity to explore the reasons for the dysfunction such as family dysfunction or early abuse. It is also an opportunity to do a great deal of teaching about nutrition. Those with dementias are particularly prone to mistake one ingredient for another or to even add nonfoods to the mixture. Care must be taken to supervise such patients closely until their functional level is assessed.

Personality-disordered patients, alcoholics and drug abusers should have little difficulty in most food preparation activities. Meals make a good opportunity to discuss how life without drugs or alcohol will affect their mealtime patterns. The mildly retarded with IQs of 50 to 70 may often live in situations where cooking for themselves is expected. Sometimes they marry and have families. Meal planning, cooking and clean-up are very important skills to be developed with this population. The moderately retarded with IQs of 35 to 50 may enjoy cooking but need careful supervision. They seldom progress beyond second grade academic skills. Few of these people marry. Often they live in group homes where food needs are filled and no cooking is necessary.[23,24]

Instructional curricula for food preparation can be purchased from the vendors listed in Appendix I.

Pediatrics

Bonding between infants and adults is most often associated with receiving and giving food. Early play experiences for children often involve playing house, making mud or sand pies and having tea parties. Early work experiences may involve feeding pets, cleaning up after themselves after meals or getting their own snack. Children do not often like highly spiced foods. Simple food preparation like stuffing celery or stirring chocolate mix into milk may be good for young children. Puppets can be an avenue for children with an eating problem to deal with feelings they have related to their illness.[24] Children eight to 12 years of age may enjoy making cookies, sandwiches or preparing frozen pizza. Teenagers often benefit from the complete preparation sequence, making a list, shopping, cooking, eating and cleaning up. Eating can be a very social time for adolescents who are attempting to decide who they are and what they value. When cooking with children or adolescents beware of food ending up on the ceiling or walls! Close supervision is recommended.[25,26]

Geriatrics

Since most of the elderly are women and traditionally women have been homemakers and cooks, many elderly patients will have a rich history of cooking on which to draw. Reminiscence groups may elicit accounts of wonderful foods prepared in the past. Actual cooking experiences sometimes elicit involvement from patients whose memory problems keep them from participation in many other activities. Somehow the stimulation of the smell and taste receptors seems to jog memories that appear otherwise unretrievable. Vision problems can interfere with reading recipes, reading package ingredients and setting oven dials. Hearing difficulties will make kitchen timers almost useless. Memory problems may cause an elderly person to forget a hot burner. Balance and arthritis difficulties can make carrying pots and ingredients hazardous. The kitchen is the most common place for accidents to happen. Nonetheless, since cooking and feeding are traditional ways to give of oneself and to oneself, this craft activity has great value for the elderly.[27-29]

Case Study

Iris is a divorced 56-year-old African-American domestic worker. She was employed by a 35-year-old single mother who was the vice-president of a mortgage company. Iris cared for the woman's child as well as her house. In her late 40s, Iris was put on hypertension and cholesterol-lowering drugs by her physician. These problems had seemed to be controlled until Iris suffered a left cardiovascular accident (CVA). After recovering from unconsciousness, she found herself unable to pull herself up off the carpet where she fell. She had to wait for her employer to return from work in the evening before she was discovered. The ambulance took her to the emergency department of a large nearby university teaching hospital. Her employer called her children to meet her at the emergency department. It was decided that immediate carotid artery surgery would help prevent further damage. After this procedure, she was placed on the neurointensive care unit.

It was here that the occupational therapist first evaluated her. He assessed her passive range of motion, active range of motion, muscle tone, strength, her oral musculature, visual-motor perception, sensory perception, cognition and general emotional mood. She was found to have right unilateral paresis in both upper and lower extremities with diminished tactile perception of sharp/dull, hot/cold, position in space and two-point perception. Her right hand had a very weak grip with some cog wheeling as she attempted to move it. Her right leg would buckle under her soon after she got onto her feet. Physical therapy began to work with her in gait training. When the occupational therapist tested her oral musculature she had some weakness though she could achieve lip closure and had no trouble swallowing.

In the interview with Iris, the occupational therapist had no difficulty understanding her responses though her speech was slow and slurred. She labored over each sentence. He found Iris to be rather depressed and worried about her job. Her employer had been paying her health insurance. She feared that her employer would find another domestic worker before Iris recovered and that she might loose her health insurance benefits as well as her job, which she liked better than any domestic job she had held before. The pay was good compared to other domestic workers' pay and her employer was concerned about her welfare. The occupational therapist told Iris he would send the social worker to help her with these issues. Iris' daughter rearranged her schedule to partially take over her mother's job while she was in the hospital. The occupational therapist and Iris discussed a kitchen evaluation to see how much she could actually do.

On the fifth day after the carotid surgery, Iris was moved out of neurointensive care onto the medical floor. At this time, the certified occupational therapy assistant (COTA) took her in a wheelchair to the occupational therapy kitchen for a screening. First the COTA showed her where things were in the kitchen. She showed Iris how easily she could roll the wheelchair up to the sink and countertop stove in the adapted kitchen. Iris slowly told her that the kitchen of her employer had high countertops and a microwave over the stove. The COTA reassured her that she would probably have more recovery before she went back to work. Indeed, it did appear that Iris had begun to have some recovery in her right hand though her leg still buckled under her. In the kitchen evaluation, the COTA asked Iris to start by making a tuna sandwich. Iris was able to wash a celery stalk but had trouble trimming it before she put it in the food processor. She had difficulty using the electric can opener. The COTA showed her several helpful techniques such as holding the bowl in her lap for mixing and using a rimmed cutting board for spreading the tuna salad on the bread.

As they worked together, Iris began to talk about her job and family life. She told of occasions when her employer had guests, of how she often made and served elaborate six-course meals. Often on these evenings, she stayed overnight at her employer's home. Her own children were grown though two still lived with her in her little house. Iris described her job as interesting and fulfilling. She had been a domestic worker most of her adult life.

She had worked five years in her present job and it had been the best job she'd ever had. She'd never felt as much as a part of a family for whom she worked as she had on her current job. Her main goal as she expressed it, was to get back to work.

After the COTA and the occupational therapist had a chance to discuss her various evaluations, they decided she would probably benefit from having all her therapy in the occupational therapy kitchen. Her sessions were scheduled at 11:30 am and the kitchen was instructed to send a tray of raw food that Iris would prepare for herself after her exercises. In the occupational therapy kitchen, everything could be reached from the wheelchair though Iris was able increasingly to pull herself up to standing if necessary. Using the over-the-sink paring board, Iris made vegetable salad, cut vegetables for a casserole and sliced fruit for gelatin salad. By the end of the second week, she was almost independent in preparing her lunch.

At this time she was transferred to the rehabilitation center in the same hospital complex. Close communication between the two occupational therapy departments made it possible for the rehabilitation occupational therapist to make a smooth transition for Iris. During her six weeks in the rehabilitation hospital she learned how to use many new pieces of adaptive equipment such as a reacher, a one-handed can opener, a jar opener, a miracle peeler and a special Swedish knife for those with weak grip. Her strength in her right hand had gradually shown improvement but was still not fully recovered. With the special Swedish knife, she was able to do almost all the cutting she needed. On her last session before being discharged, Iris cooked a meal for the occupational therapy staff as her way of saying thank you. She made oven-barbecued ribs, field peas, turnip greens and corn bread. The only assistance she had had was with shelling the peas. She got a paraplegic patient to help her with that as she still had some problems with some fine motor activities. The occupational therapy staff helped her serve the meal. Most of Iris' initial depression was gone and on this occasion was not evident at all.

Iris started back to her job on a part-time basis. She moved into the guest room at her employer's house so she would not have to deal immediately with taking the city bus. Initially she just cooked the evening meal and supervised the child when she returned from school. At the end of seven months, Iris was working full-time again.

Discussion Questions

1. If the CVA victim in the case study was a male laborer, not a female, how could cooking be adapted to appeal to him?
2. If a member of a cooking group has special dietary needs such as salt-free meals or a strict diabetic diet, how could you adapt meal planning and cooking of spaghetti to fill his or her needs?
3. Patients taking the kind of antidepressant drug called "MAO Inhibitors" are prohibited from eating the following foods because they could cause a hypertensive crisis:
   - Beans
   - Aged cheese
   - Yeast
   - Beer
   - Liquor
   - Wine
   - Yogurt
   - Liver
   - Pickled herring

   Plan a menu and choose recipes safe for such a patient.

References

1. Webster's Seventh New Collegiate Dictionary. (1969). Springfield, MA: G & C Merriam Company.
2. Beeuwkes, A.M., Todhunter, E.H., & Weigley, E.S. (Eds.). (1967). *Essays on History of Nutrition and Dietetics*. Chicago: The American Dietetics Association.

3. Ritchie, C.I.A. (1981). *Food in Civilization.* Sydney, Australia: Methuen Australia Pty., Ltd.

4. Hames, C.C. & Joseph, D.H. (1986). *Basic Concepts of Helping: A Holistic Approach,* 2nd ed. Norwalk, CT: Appleton-Century-Crofts.

5. Hamilton, E.M. & Whitney, E. (1979). *Nutrition Concepts and Controversies.* St. Paul, MN: West Publishing Company.

6. Mosey, A.C. (1986). *Psychosocial Components of Occupational Therapy.* New York: Raven Press.

7. Colson, J.H.C. (1944). *The Rehabilitation of the Injured: Occupational Therapy.* London: Cassell and Company.

8. Dunton, W.R. & Licht, S. (1957). *Occupational Therapy Principles and Practice.* Springfield, IL: Charles C. Thomas.

9. Fidler, G.S. & Fidler, J.W. (1954). *Introduction to Psychiatric Occupational Therapy.* New York: The MacMillan Co.

10. Hall, H.J. & Buck, M.M.C. (1916). *Handicrafts for the Handicapped.* New York: Moffat, Yard and Co.

11. Willard, H.S. & Spackman, C.E. (1947). *Principles of Occupational Therapy.* Philadelphia: Lippincott.

12. Hopkins, H.L. & Smith, H.D. (1988). *Willard and Spackman's Occupational Therapy,* 7th ed. Philadelphia: Lippincott.

13. Hopkins, H.L. & Smith, H.D. (1978). *Willard and Spackman's Occupational Therapy,* 5th ed. Philadelphia: Lippincott.

14. MacDonald, E.M. (1960). *Occupational Therapy in Rehabilitation.* London: Bailliere, Tindall and Cox.

15. Trombly, C.A. (1983). *Occupational Therapy for Physical Dysfunction,* 2nd ed. Baltimore: Waverly Press.

16. Jacobs, K. (1985). *Occupational Therapy: Work-Related Programs and Assessments.* Boston: Little, Brown.

17. Hemphill, B.J. (1988). *Mental Health Assessment in Occupational Therapy.* Thorofare, NJ: Slack.

18. Kane, R.A. & Kane, R.L. (1985). *Assessing the Elderly: A Practical Guide to Measurement.* Lexington, MA: Lexington Books.

19. Early, M.B. (1987). *Mental Health Concepts and Techniques for the Occupational Therapy Assistant.* New York: Raven Press.

20. Practice Division. (1988). *Mental Health Information Packet.* Rockville, MD: American Occupational Therapy Association.

21. Hershey Pasta Group Kitchens. (1985). *The Hurry Up I'm Hungry Pasta Cookbook.* Hershey, PA: Hershey Foods Corporation.

22. Hopkins, H.L. & Smith, H.D. (1988). *Willard and Spackman's Occupational Therapy,* 7th ed. Philadelphia: Lippincott.

23. American Psychiatric Association. (1987). *Diagnostic and Statistical Manual of Mental Disorders,* 3rd ed., revised. Washington, DC: American Psychiatric Association, Author.

24. Robinson, N.M. & Robinson, H.B. (1976). *The Mentally Retarded Child: A Psychological Approach.* New York: McGraw-Hill.

25. Saunders, F.M. (1987). *Your Diabetic Child.* New York: Bantam Books.

26. Pratt, P.N. & Allen, A.S. (1989). *Occupational Therapy for Children,* 2nd ed. St. Louis: Mosby.

27. Desnick, S.G. (1971). *Geriatric Contentment.* Springfield, IL: Charles C. Thomas.

28. Mace, N.L. & Robins, P.V. (1981). *The 36-Hour Day.* Baltimore: Johns Hopkins University Press.

29. Wolff, K. (1970). *The Emotional Rehabilitation of the Geriatric Patient.* Springfield, IL: Charles C. Thomas.

15
Computer Art as a Craft

▼

Introduction

Initially, it is important to say what this chapter is not. It is not going to tell how to buy a computer, what kind to buy, how to use it, how to speak computerese/computer jargon or what the computer's potential for total patient treatment could be. There are some good books about this already.[1-5] Remember, though, that the computer field, like all technologies, is constantly being improved and refined.

It is hard to pinpoint the first computer. Some say it was the abacus, which is 2,500 years old.[6] Others say it was a primitive slide-rule-type machine invented in Germany in 1623.[7] In this century, B.F. Skinner, the American father of behavioral therapy and of teaching machines, has been given credit as a pioneer in this field. His 1953 effort to help his daughter with arithmetic with a machine using cards, levers and lights may have been the grandparent of today's modern computer graphics.[8]

In occupational therapy, the first articles on computers and occupational therapy appeared in the 1960s.[9] The 1973 article in *The American Journal of Occupational Therapy*, "Computers and Occupational Therapy,"[10] mentions art and recreation as possible therapy tools. "In the year 2000 . . . everyone will be a graphics user" according to Thomas Kucharvy.[11] However, just as crafts cannot be replaced, so computers will not eliminate our other treatment modalities. They are just additional tools.[9]

Bedside computer terminals for acute care hospitals are being predicted for the next decade. Their primary purpose will be for record keeping and documentation of the patient's condition. However, if a bedside terminal is available, therapists could use it for patient treatment. In the same way in which a therapist sometimes allows patients to continue to work on an occupational therapy project on their own after the therapist has left, so patients might be allowed to keep computer software and work on it at their leisure.[12]

In the same developmental way that children naturally draw before they write, most adults could use graphics before learning word processing. Many graphics software packages make simple lines and shapes that are the first marks besides scribbles that children make when they begin to handle pencils and crayons. Other software allows the user to simply color in existing pictures. Software programs are on a soft floppy plastic disk. When a person, even a therapist, first attempts to draw using a mouse, which is the usual hand control for graphics, it is similar to the experience a child has when first starting to use writing implements. The mouse responds to the users untrained hand in which a tiny muscle contraction sends the pencil cursor on the screen streaking off in an unintended direction.

Some patients may have or will develop more skill and creative possibilities with graphics software while others may benefit from and enjoy programs in which pictures are predrawn. The patient needs only to choose the picture, which can then be rotated, stretched or changed in size. This spectrum of available graphics software makes it possible to easily grade the activity up or down. Computer graphics are similar to painting in which for some patients, paint-by-number is appropriate and for others, oil paint motivates them to create. Truly, computer art can be a helpful craft for patients who think of themselves as being a part of our modern computer age. Other arts, such as poetry writing, music composition and arrangement can be done on the computer. The idea of creating with this technology can be truly motivating for some patients.

Frequency of Use

Few clinics have computers that can be made available for patient treatment. However, this is rapidly changing. While most clinics use their computers for record keeping and cognitive evaluations, the use of computers for treatment is becoming more commonplace. Therapists choose computers to accomplish various treatment objectives: to improve cognition, increase fine motor control and encourage self-expression. As more clinics acquire computers and computer expertise, it will increase as a treatment activity.

Assessments

Computer assessments in occupational therapy include various kinds of evaluations, not all of which are graphic. Graphic means pictorial arts or clear visual images. Cognitive dysfunction, which includes attention deficits, memory problems, confusion, lack of comprehension and judgment, and decreased ability to problem solve is one of the areas most often evaluated using computers.

Graphics are used in evaluation of head-injured and learning-disabled patients.[13] Initially, patients must be evaluated for appropriateness of computer assessment. Can they see the screen well enough? Can they manipulate the implements to give commands to the computer? Can they comprehend the instructions and questions asked by the computer? Graphics can be used to evaluate patients for vocational appropriateness for drafting or similar careers.[13] A game called Gremlin Hunt can be used for assessment in head injury and with the developmentally disabled. The graphics are attractive and colorful and appropriate for patients eight years of age and up.[14] For patients with perceptual problems, Visual Organization software evaluates figure ground and missing parts.[15] Early and Advanced Switch Games can be used in either treatment or evaluation in using graphics to complete pictures, match shapes and colors, and for directionality and motor planning. The Early Games are for children up through sixth grade. The Advance Games are for people up through tenth grade.[16]

The computer is absolutely objective and cannot be manipulated as a therapist can. This can be valuable in evaluating some kinds of patients.

Main Therapeutic Applications

Physical Dysfunction

There are some devices that help the physically disabled patient do computer graphics. A joy stick is a hand-operated stick control that can move the cursor over the screen to give commands. A light-pencil control can be used by aiming the lighted end of the pencil on the screen to give commands. Another aid is the paddle control used in computer games. A paddle control is a board, usually with two hand-held switches that control the action on the screen for two-player games such as tennis, hockey and squash (Figure 15-1). A paddle can also be plugged into a regular television set. These games use graphics or pictures rather than words. Such controls allow patients with severely restricted upper extremity and body movements to control the pictures on the screen. Some games and graphics can be slowed for the restricted user.[17] Patients with physical problems who could benefit from computer craft are those who suffer from spinal cord injury, multiple sclerosis and Guillian-Barre. They can use these games to increase motor control.

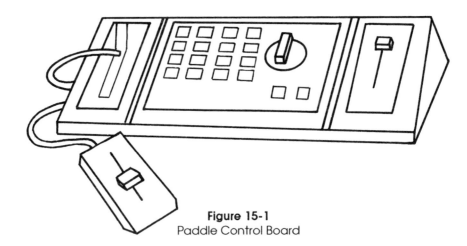

Figure 15-1
Paddle Control Board

As with assessment, those physical dysfunction patients with cognitive problems are often good candidates for use of computer graphics in treatment. These patients may have acquired their cognitive deficits from many different causes, such as developmental problems, cerebrovascular accident, head injury, cerebral palsy or learning disabilities.[18,19]

Mental Health

High-functioning patients can benefit from working with innovative graphics. Concentration, attention span and fatigue, which are frequent problems for depressed patients, could all be addressed through this medium. Manic patients would need precautions as their hyperactivity, impatience and poor impulse control could make this activity frustrating. Also they could damage expensive hardware in their excessive movement. This should only be used with manic patients who have been stabilized on psychotropic medication. Cognition, such as thinking and problem solving, may be difficult activities for some schizophrenics. A schizophrenic patient who could benefit might be in a daycare or sheltered workshop program but would be unlikely to be found in more acute treatment situations. Patients with personality disorders may find computer work appealing as their cognitive and perceptual-motor functions are usually intact unless they have been damaged through abuse of drugs or alcohol. Few mentally retarded have the creative capacity to use the more sophisticated drawing programs; however, the higher-functioning retarded patients may enjoy the packages with predrawn pictures. Some of the children's shape and design programs could be helpful in working with the mentally retarded. The therapist would need to be careful that such graphics were not perceived as kid stuff by the retarded person, thus making the graphics not age appropriate. In all cases, the success of using graphics would be volitional. Motivation for using the computer may be the single most important reason to use it with psychiatric patients.[17]

Pediatrics

Pediatric patients may be the best candidates for computer treatment as they have often already been exposed to computers if they are of school age.[20] They do not have the inherent fear and mental block about new technology that older patients often have. Originally there had been fears that computer use by children would cause them to fail to develop social skills and to become withdrawn. This appears to have been an exaggerated alarm. Children have grown up being constantly exposed to television and apparently have learned to be perceptive of what comes on the screen in a way that older people have not. Consequently, they are often more able to learn from designs and pictures on a computer monitor, which resembles a television screen, than are older patients. An added benefit is that computers give immediate, nonjudgmental, reliable feedback to children about their actions and behavior. Computers cannot be manipulated as adult humans can.

Geriatrics

This patient population may be least likely to benefit from computer graphics. Many elders have slowed in their thought processes and movements. The very basis of computing is speed and efficiency, the opposite of what many elders want to do. They want to be allowed to move and think more slowly. In our culture we allow them that prerogative.

Diminished eyesight is often a problem for geriatric patients. Computer screens are sometimes difficult to focus on visually for more than a few minutes. While we may get the occasional alert older patient who is used to operating a computer, it is not common. Graphics may be a new challenge for such a patient.

O'Leary, Mann and Perashki[21] discuss problems older people have with the use of computers and offer some solutions related to positioning, vision, strength and cognition. They provide an extensive list of resources for adaptive computer equipment.

Case Study

Emily is a ten-year-old severely contracted cerebral palsy patient. It was unknown until she was eight years old that she had an IQ of 110. Because she was so physically handicapped and her language was limited, and because there was no one trained to test her IQ by non-pencil-and-paper methods before, it was thought that she was retarded as well as physically limited. Emily was of African-American and Puerto Rican heritage and was born in New York City. At age two and one-half years, her mother had moved with her back to her home in the South. Shortly thereafter, her mother, who had been a drug addict, died of an overdose. Emily was taken to live with her grandmother in a rural community. She had had no schooling except what she saw on television. When Emily was eight, the grandmother died and no one else in the family was willing to care for Emily, as she required total personal care, feeding, diapering and bathing.

The state child welfare agency made a decision to place her in an intermediate care facility for the developmentally disabled. She was finally evaluated and measured for her own wheelchair. At this time she was enrolled in a special education class. She was evaluated by all the members of the treatment team. At that time her IQ was discovered to be 110. A concerted effort was made by all the professions involved with Emily to help her make up for the time when she had had no schooling. Her upper extremity athetosis made most occupational activities difficult for her. The occupational therapy goals were to:

- Increase self-care such as self-feeding, learning to sit on the toilet and control the timing of toileting;
- Learn visual and perceptual motor skills;
- Enhance and stimulate visual acuity;
- Improve upper extremity fine motor coordination; and
- Develop a feeling of independence and autonomy.

She was evaluated for appropriateness of computer use. The therapist found that Emily could begin to control the screen by using a joy stick on her wheelchair lap board. A program was begun with the school teacher working with Emily to learn to read. She had taught herself some words by simply watching television. While attending occupational therapy, she worked with the computer graphics as a reward for feeding herself and for waiting to sit on the toilet to urinate and defecate. She started out with a simple program of lines and shapes that she could color in and move around the screen. But she rapidly advanced to a more sophisticated program involving assembling designs on the screen. The therapist worked with her on visually scanning her work, developing figure ground perception by seeing shapes within shapes and figures, on color discrimination and sequencing her actions to get the effects she wanted, and from there to drawing and painting on more sophisticated software. The occupational therapy clinic did not have a color printer so the therapist sent her floppy disk to the curriculum center at the board of education building to have the graphics printed out from Emily's drawings. Soon Emily was skilled enough to draw her own cartoons which she used on greeting cards.

The school staff used her enlarged cartoons for signs and warnings around the school building. Emily was seen as a good candidate for a new group home for the disabled that was going to be funded by a grant. The occupational therapist worked with the grant writers to see that money was included to buy computers for each resident's room.

Discussion Questions

1. How could the possibility of increasing Emily's social isolation be avoided as she became more involved with the computer?
2. Could any of the movements she learned to make with the joy stick be transferred over to help her in increasing her independence in self-care?

References

1. Clark, E.N. (1986). *Microcomputers: Clinical Applications.* Thorofare, NJ: Slack.
2. Cromwell, F.S. (1986). *Computer Applications in Occupational Therapy.* New York: The Haworth Press.
3. McWilliams, P. (1984). *Personal Computers and the Disabled.* Garden City, NY: Doubleday and Company.
4. Practice Division. (1985). *Computers: Information Packet.* Rockville, MD: American Occupational Therapy Association.
5. Ryan, S. (Ed.). (1986). *The Certified Occupational Therapy Assistant: Roles and Responsibilities.* Thorofare, NJ: Slack.
6. Pascoe, L.C. (1974). *Encyclopedia of Dates and Events.* Kent, United Kingdom: Hadder and Stroughton, Ltd.
7. Ritchie, D. (1986). *The Computer Pioneers: The Making of the Modern Computer.* New York: Simon and Schuster.
8. Hall, E. (1983). A cure for American education. *Psychology Today,* 17(9), 26-27.
9. Practice Division. (1985). *Computers: Information Packet.* Rockville, MD: American Occupational Therapy Association.
10. English, C.B. (1973). Computers and occupational therapy. *The American Journal of Occupational Therapy,* 29(1), 43-47.
11. Hallisey, J. (1989). The future is graphic. *PC Computing,* 2(7), 52.
12 American Occupational Therapy Association. (1988). In focus. *The American Journal of Occupational Therapy,* 42 (May)(9): 615.
13. Milner, D. (1984). Use of a microcomputer in treatment of patients with physical disabilities. *Physical Disabilities Special Interest Section Newsletter,* 7(2), 1-3.
14. Timms, J. (1989). Software and technology reviews. *American Journal of Occupational Therapy,* 43(4), 267.
15. Redding, K. (1991). Software and technology reviews. *American Journal of Occupational Therapy,* 45(6), 569-570.
16. Dilly, S.K. (February, 1990). Software & technology reviews. *American Journal of Occupational Therapy,* 44(2), 179.
17. Clark, E.N. (1986). *Microcomputers: Clinical Applications.* Thorofare, NJ: Slack.
18. Gracey, S. (1984). Computer assisted therapy for brain injured patients: A team approach. *Physical Disabilities Special Interest Section Newsletter,* 7(2): 4.
19. Skinner, A.D. & Trachtman, L.H. (1985). Brief or new: Use of the computer program (PC Coloring Book in Cognitive Rehabilitation). *American Journal of Occupational Therapy,* 39(7), 470-471.
20. Levin, G. (1985). Computers and kids: The good news. *Psychology Today,* 19(8), 50-51.
21. O'Leary, Mann, C., & Perkash, I. (1991). Access to computers for older adults: Problems and solutions. *American Journal of Occupational Therapy,* 45(7), 636-642.

16

Art Techniques: Drawing and Painting

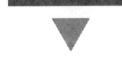

Introduction

Drawing may be the oldest craft used for healing about which we know. While the crafts discussed so far in this book may be old, it was not until the last few centuries that they have been used in healing. Drawing has been used for millenia in healing practices and other rituals that attempt to control nature.[1,2]

Before humans had any knowledge of anatomy and physiology, images conceived in the brain and drawn on the wall were considered as real as any other product such as a slingshot and were believed to have as much real power. Images were integral in both killing and healing rituals. The Greeks carried on these practices in the temples of Aesculapias. However, the 17th century French philosopher René Descartes emphasized the mind-body split. This reinforced a direction in which medicine was already headed, that the mind and body were separate and needed different healing treatments. Emotions did not qualify as having any relation to disease.[3]

In the 19th century in Switzerland, the force of imagery began to be studied in earnest by psychologists. Freud was aware of the power of imagery in treatment though he seldom used it himself.[4] Florence Goodenough published her work on drawing as an intelligence test in 1926. Art therapy began to develop in the 1920s in the same era that occupational therapy had its start.[5,6] Art therapists specialized in using art in healing. Occupational therapists have used drawing, in the same way as they have used so many other activities, when it was the best activity to help rehabilitate a patient to functioning most independently. The first issue of Willard and Spackman's *Occupational Therapy*[7] has a section on drawing and sketching in treatment. It focuses on both physical and mental as well as pediatric uses of art. About this same time, those researching the meaning of drawings began to publish their findings.[8-11] While drawing and painting have never been the major modalities in occupational therapy as they are in art therapy, occupational therapists have felt free to use these activities when they were the best ones for the patient. These are important techniques for occupational therapists to keep in their armamentarium of treatment tools.

Frequency of Use

Fingerpainting is used in one-fourth to one-half of all clinics. Fingerpainting is used to provide an outlet for frustration, to encourage self-expression to increase sensory input and to improve bilateral dexterity. Painting with watercolors, acrylics or oils is an activity often used to improve fine motor control and eye-hand coordination. Drawing with pencils or crayons occurs in almost half the clinics. Drawing is often used to improve group socialization, to improve fine motor control, to encourage self-expression and to improve self-concept.

Assessments

There are more drawing assessments than any other craft or art media. Perhaps this is because it is so simple to ask for a drawing that requires few materials, and that can be done almost anywhere with individuals or groups. Drawing is adaptable to almost any assessment situation. Many of the assessments mentioned here were developed by occupational therapists in the 1960s and 1970s when the profession was concentrating on standardizing administration, observations and analyses of task behavior. The first three described below are often used by other professions as well, such as psychology. Perhaps the House-Tree-Person test is one of the earliest drawing assessments[12] that is still used. Except for the standard request to draw a house, a tree and a person, on 8 1/2in. by 11in. white paper, this is an unstructured test. The order of drawing is theorized to move from the least threatening, the house, to most threatening symbol, the person. There are guidelines for interpreting each drawing.[13]

The Goodenough-Harris Drawing Test is for children ages three to 15 years and can be used individually or in a group. The children are asked to draw first a man, then a woman and last, themselves. There is a scoring guide that tells how to look at each separate item: head, neck, nose, etc. The scores show the child's functioning in relation to age performance expectations.[10]

The Draw-a-Person Catalog for Interpretive Analysis[14] is unstructured. Patients are simply told to draw a person any way they like. The picture is discussed afterward with the therapist. The catalog has lists of warnings and abnormality indicators for body parts as well as drawing quality. There are a number of checklist forms to assist in documenting the assessment.

The Azima Battery, which was first developed in the late 1950s and early 1960s, includes a free or unstructured drawing, a drawing of a person of the same and opposite sex, an unstructured clay project and fingerpainting. It is for use in psychiatric occupational therapy. It is intended to assess awareness of reality, perceptions of others, mood, energy level and ego defenses.[15]

The Diagnostic Test Battery has five tasks: drawing, ceramics, painting, woodwork and leather. It was intended to be for adult psychiatric patients. The House-Tree-Person test is used for the drawing portion. The painting part of the test is an unstructured water color. Assessment findings should be expected to include expressiveness, compulsiveness, cognitive processes, mood and approach to task.[16]

The Fidler Diagnostic Battery was developed in the early 1960s for use with individual clients. It included drawing, fingerpainting and working with clay. This was refined and developed into the Activity Laboratory that could be used with groups of patients. The Activity Laboratory also has three activities: cutting out and coloring a stencil, fingerpainting and assembling a collage. The sequence from structured to unstructured tasks is intended to demonstrate how the patient deals with limits. The group setting helps look at social skills. Fine motor performance is also observed.[15]

The O'Kane Diagnostic Battery for Psychiatry is projective in nature. There are three charcoal drawings, three fingerpaintings and a clay project. The administration is structured.[17]

The Kinetic Family Drawing is normed for ages five to 20 years. Patients are simply asked to draw the people in their family. The manual has pictures of patient drawings and discussion of a wide variety of symbols and situations. Some therapists incorporate a more informal version of this assessment into a battery of other evaluations in pediatric psychiatry.[18]

The Goodman Battery includes a free or unstructured drawing, a drawing of a person along with a tile task and clay work. This assessment looks at approach to task, affect, impulsiveness, compulsiveness, organization and symbolic content. It is for adolescents and adults.[15]

The Copy Flower House Test is a subjective assessment that is included in a battery for evaluating a variety of perceptual problems experienced by stroke patients. Unilateral neglect is specifically assessed by the two drawings of a flower and a house. Informal person drawings are also helpful in working with patients who have suffered a cerebrovascular accident (CVA) for evaluation of body visualization and somatogenosia.[19]

The Bay Area Functional Performance Evaluation (BaFPE) for psychiatry, for patients aged 16 years and older, has five tasks and an assessment of a patient's social skills. The five tasks are shell sorting, check depositing, drawing a house plan, arranging a block pattern and drawing a person doing something. This test is well-validated and though scoring is initially difficult to learn, it provides good data on dysfunctional areas. Research continues on the BaFPE. It has been revised several times since its introduction in 1978-1979.[17]

The BH Battery has a tile task and fingerpainting. While the materials arrangement is structured, the instructions to the patient for painting are not. The patient is timed and the manual provides a rating scale for each activity. Documentation for this assessment is oriented toward behavioral description rather than content analysis.[20]

In the Mattis' Dementia Rating Scale, patients are asked to draw a self-portrait, a picture of a person sitting across from them, a face, a house and a simple still life of arranged objects. This evaluation, developed by an art therapist, is used in helping diagnose dementia. Perceptual deficits such as figure collision and confusion may indicate dementia.[21]

The Gross Activity Battery has three projective activities: charcoal drawing, fingerpainting and working with clay. The administration is highly structured as is the way in which it is reported. It can be used with any age or patient population.[17]

The Elizur Test of Psycho-Organicity: Children and Adults is a 10-minute test for individuals aged six years and up. The purpose is to differentiate the patients with organic brain problems from those without. The test uses drawings, digits and blocks.[17]

Many checklists of leisure preference such as the Neuropsychiatric Interest (NPI) Checklist include painting or drawing. These sorts of art techniques offer good potential for leisure activities for many people.[22] A person does not have to be an artist to enjoy making art.

Supplies

It is not necessary to have an elaborate supply of art materials to have success in using drawing and painting for crafts. The following materials and supplies are adequate for most clinics.

Twelve- by 18in. paper is best for most art projects as it allows enough room to draw freely without taking up too much table space. The following types should be kept available for artwork:
- Newsprint paper—12in. by 18in.;
- White drawing paper—12in. by 18in.;

- Manila paper—12in. by 18in.; and
- Fingerpaint paper—16in. by 22in.

Patients can share boxes of crayons and pens, thus increasing social skills while requiring fewer individual sets of colors.

- #2 pencils with erasers;
- Crayons;
- Chalk or chalk pastels;
- Oil pastels;
- Felt-tip markers;
- Powdered tempra paint (this can be mixed with dish detergent and water to make fingerpaint);
- Boxes of watercolors with semi-moist half pans; and
- An assortment of brushes.

In special instances, oil paints may be desirable for patients who are artists. Otherwise, watercolor or tempra is adequate for most painting projects.

Drawing and Painting

There is such a vast array of techniques for using drawing and painting in therapy, that the development of a separate profession, art therapy, was natural in the same way that the diversity of plant-growing techniques made horticulture therapy natural. Occupational therapy incorporates aspects of both into treatment when the situation indicates.[23-25] Apart from the evaluations discussed before, occupational therapists use many art media to achieve patient goals. Several are described below.

Murals

Murals are a way of using art to achieve a group goal. A mural can be drawn with crayons or painted with tempra paint. They can be done on brown butcher paper, on glass windows at holidays or on newsprint. Sometimes newspaper publishers have the ends of rolls of newsprint that they cannot use and may be willing to donate. This paper is good for group murals. Painting on windows is fun until it is time to clean them off. The work involved in removal can be minimized by adding liquid detergent to the tempra paints when mixing them. Damp rags will often remove this paint with less effort. Liquid dish detergent added to tempra paints gives a nice consistency to the paint as well as allowing it to wash out of clothing more easily. If brown butcher paper is used, tempra paint is bright enough to overcome the darkness of the brown background. It is difficult to make crayon show up on brown butcher paper. It is better to use bright felt markers on it instead, if drawing is to be used rather than painting.

Crayon Resist
This technique elevates crayons to a more sophisticated level for most patients.

PROCESS
1. Using 12in. x 18in. manila paper, have the patient draw a crayon design or picture with white or pale pastel colors.
2. Put one drop of water in the half-pan of watercolor to be used. Allow the water to soften the color for a few minutes. It is better to use a bright vivid color to contrast with the crayon.
3. Dip the brush into the water and stroke the top of the watercolor half-pan to gather color into the brush. Then apply the watercolor to the whole sheet.
4. Repeat the softening process if necessary. This technique makes attractive snow scenes.

Crayon Etching
Crayon etching is a more difficult technique and requires physical effort and endurance but usually produces an attractive product. Use paper with a tooth, which means slightly rough, such as construction or manila paper. It may be best to start with a smaller size at first such as 8 1/2in. x 11in.

PROCESS
1. Heavily color all areas of the paper with different colors. It works well if the colors are in sections of contrasting colors. Color heavily to make sure none of the paper shows through.
2. Use a black crayon to completely cover all the other colors.
3. When no color shows through the black, use a sharp instrument like the pointed end of a leather tracing modeler to scratch a picture through the black crayon.

This activity can use up a lot of energy and aggression, because of the effort involved coloring in and scratching through the surface. This classifies as a constructive/destructive craft in which a patient can sublimate negative impulses. This kind of activity can use motions that simulate destructive force at the same time the patient is creating.

Main Therapeutic Applications

Physical Dysfunction
Fingerpainting may be used with a patient who is working on motion of the hand and arm. Because the paint reduces the friction between hand and paper, it is easier to get movement.

Painting with a brush can be a prewriting exercise for a patient with hand injury. The brush handle can be built up with cylindrical foam padding for patients with arthritis, hand patients or for those with weakened grip. Because watercolor requires little strength, it is an appropriate activity for someone who is very weak. Tempra and water color wash out of cloth easily and will not permanently stain bed clothes.[26]

Mental Health

Art techniques are most often used with psychiatric patients. These media allow for expression of most feelings. Color, texture, patterns and spacing can all be used to express emotions for the patient. What the patient says while working should be remembered and noted on the back of the artwork. This is frequently helpful to the psychiatrist and other staff members. Art offers many opportunities for patients to focus on problem areas. Working together in a room with other patients gives the patient the opportunity to practice social skills.

Pediatrics

Drawing preceeds writing as a way of expression. Young children start by making lines, then scribbles, circles with arms and legs and facial features, and then other shapes. Some feel that developmental maturation is easily visible in children's drawings. Thick kindergarten crayons are best for young children as they have not developed enough fine motor control to use regular crayons. With children, art is often the quickest way to see what is happening within them emotionally. They have not yet learned to censor their expression. The simplest materials—crayons, fingerpaint or tempra paint with a brush—are often better than using complicated techniques. Young children need larger paper, 18in. x 24in., as they have more difficulty with fine motor control. Manual dexterity can be improved with painting and drawing. The experience of art is usually so much fun for young children, that they are seldom critical of the product.

Older children often enjoy the different techniques such as crayon resist or crayon etching. Their hand control is usually adequate to accomplish the realism that children attempt in their art from ages eight to 12 years. Colored pencils are often enjoyed by this age group.[10,27,28]

Adolescents are usually self-conscious about their art. This can be minimized by doing abstract art, which allows them to avoid the self-consciousness about their ability to draw realistically. They can enjoy patterns and new techniques that allow them to focus on the art rather than their drawing skill.

Geriatrics

The first response that many older people give to requests that they participate in art activities is often "I can't draw." Crafts that involve art such as tole painting or stencils may assist in easing older adults into art. It is important to use sophisticated adult materials like pen and ink rather than child-oriented materials like crayons. Playing classical music during the activity has been found to counteract older adults feeling of being involved in a childish activity. Drawings and paintings offer older adults wonderful opportunities to reminisce. A therapist can help them focus on their own life by asking them to draw simple life experiences, by asking them to draw simple things from their childhood or young adult life: food, tools, clothes, pets and flowers. Many people are phobic about drawing human figures or faces. These could be incorporated into later sessions. Drawing memories provides an opportunity for older people to make peace with their life while they preserve it for others through pictures. Elders may want to share their art works with grandchildren as a way of showing "this is how it was back then."[29]

Case Study

Danny was a 42-year-old third-generation Japanese-American dock worker. While unloading a ship his right arm was smashed and had to be amputated. He was right handed. He had an above-the-elbow amputation. This was a very traumatic event for Danny as he had been earning his living by using his hands since he was 16 years old. His parents had run a small neighborhood grocery store and Danny had worked in the store as far back as he could remember until he quit high school in his junior year. He took a job with his uncle on his fishing boat. At age 22, in 1968, he joined the Navy. During his four-year enlistment, he met men from everywhere. He worked on his GED (general education diploma) and completed it. It was his hope to attend college when he was discharged from the service. When he got home, he had difficulty adjusting to shore life in the same way other Vietnam veterans had trouble adapting to civilian life. His childhood sweetheart got pregnant so they got married. He took a job working on the docks. The union pay was good though the work was hard and he had never envisioned himself as a laborer. Four children came within eight years and his view of himself as a man with responsibilities dimmed his youthful dreams.

The occupational therapist visited Danny for the first time five days after the surgery. He was sitting on his bed just staring at the television set, which was showing a soap opera. It was obvious that he was not paying attention, just staring at the screen. He wore his pajama top over the bandaged stump so it was not immediately apparent which was the affected arm. Danny responded slowly and minimally to the therapist's introduction and explanation of the occupational therapy process he could expect. She asked Danny to remove his shirt and move his shoulder so she could see if he had any movement restriction. Though she could see that the stump was swollen even above the bandage, he appeared to have full range of motion. She unwrapped the stump to look at its condition. There was the normal redness where the flap was stitched. She checked his range-of-motion again and rewrapped the stump. They talked briefly about Danny's job because he assumed she would help him with employment. She explained her role in his total rehabilitation. Though she knew he had been told all this before, she also knew from a discussion of Danny's case at grand rounds that he was very depressed and confused. She knew that depressed people often forget what they have been told so she felt it was a good idea to explain each team member's role again. She discussed the necessity of a program to learn one-handed skills. Danny's response was lukewarm.

The next day after range-of-motion exercises, she had Danny hold a pencil and write his name with his left hand. She began to ask him about his experiences in writing. He told of attending Japanese school in the Buddhist temple on Saturdays as a child. As they discussed this, he remembered having learned brush calligraphy. Sometimes the teacher had given lessons on sumi-e, Japanese ink painting. He had enjoyed that. They had sometimes carried the ink and brushes outside and painted objects in the temple garden. For a moment as they talked, it seemed he had forgotten his plight. The therapist took advantage of his more animated description and asked if he might like to try to do some ink painting again during his rehabilitation. His face fell as he looked where his right hand should have been. He just shook his head. The occupational therapist said "Well, you need to begin to practice using that left hand. Let's try it." Danny looked crestfallen but he didn't say no.

The therapist had to go to the Japanese variety store to purchase rice paper, bamboo brushes and preground liquid sumi-e ink. The next day she carried these along with a pair of lefthanded scissors and the book, *The Living Art of Ink Painting*[30] into the room. Danny appeared as depressed as at the first visit, but she matter of factly put him through his exercises, his self-care training and then assisted him in unrolling the rice paper, in cutting off a piece and in opening the ink bottle. She directed him to paint his name with his left hand. He slowly picked up the brush and dipped it into the ink. As he applied the brush to the paper, it began to make a big spot where the brush touched. "I can't do this" he said. The occupational therapist reminded him that everything took practice. She left him trying his name for the third time.

The next day when she came back, he was sitting straighter. He showed her a piece of rice paper cut rather jaggedly with his name in English and Japanese calligraphy. He appeared proud of the work as he described his father's visit last evening and how his father had demonstrated what he could remember of calligraphy. They seemed to be able to talk about Japanese ink painting in a way they had been unable to share since Danny was a little boy. He said he thought he'd practice on it some more since that was what he always told his children about homework-practice. His temporary prosthesis was not fine tuned enough for him to attempt to paint with it. A few weeks later, however, when his permanent prosthesis had been fitted, the therapist began to work with him on using the bamboo sumi-e brush with his hook. She built up the handle so it was easier to grip. His first paintings were large figures, leaves and fish because he was using gross shoulder motions (Figure 16-1). It was discouraging at first as he felt he had no control. Often he also complained of phantom pain during the sessions. Gradually, his paintings began to show more refinement. Nonetheless, he began to prefer painting with his left hand rather than using the prosthesis.

The social worker worked with the Department of Vocational Rehabilitation and the union steward. They were able to get the shipping company that owned the dock where Danny worked to train him to do computer inventories of ship contents so he could return to full-time active employment rather than receiving disability money.

His renewed interest in Japanese calligraphy and art was shared by his family. As he became more skilled, one of his childhood friends who taught Japanese language in the Saturday Japanese School got him to teach an occasional class on sumi-e. By this time he was able to grind his own ink and paint in a true traditional way, using both his right prosthesis and left hand.

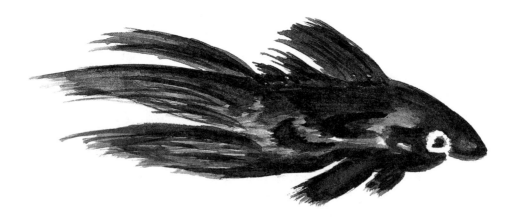

Figure 16-1
Sumi-e Painting of a Fish

Discussion Questions

1. Cultural crafts can sometimes be used to motivate patients to attempt activities. What might be an appropriate cultural craft for an Italian? A Native American? a Central American? a Scandinavian?
2. If you were planning a session with a group mural, how would you assist patients to choose a theme? How could you help them to avoid the situation in which everyone is allowed to work on any space they like thus producing a fragmented effect?
3. In which other crafts you have studied so far could drawing and painting be used? How?

References

1. Janson, H.W. (1969). *History of Art*, 2nd ed. Englewood Cliffs, NJ: Prentice Hall.
2. Lewin, R. (1988). *In the Age of Mankind*. Washington DC: Smithsonian Books.
3. Achterberg, J. (1985). *Imagery in Healing*. Boston: New Science Library.
4. Kaplan, H.I. & Sadock, B.J. (1981). *Modern Synopsis of Comprehensive Textbook of Psychiatry III*, 3rd ed. Baltimore: Williams & Wilkins.
5. Detre, K.C., et al. (1983). Roots of art therapy. *American Journal of Art Therapy*, 20(4), 111-123.
6. Ulman, E. & Dachinger, P. (Eds.). (1975). *Art Therapy in Theory and Practice*. New York: Schocken Books.
7. Willard, H.S. & Spackman, C.S. (1947). *Principles of Occupational Therapy*. Philadelphia: Lippincott.
8. Betensky, M. (1973). *Self-Discovery Through Self-Expression*. Springfield, IL: Charles C. Thomas.
9. Hammer, E.F. (1958). *The Clinical Application of Projective Drawings*. Springfield, IL: Charles C. Thomas.
10. Harris, D.B. (1963). *Children's Drawings as Measures of Intellectual Maturity*. New York: Harcourt, Brace and World Inc.
11. Machover, K. (1949). *Personality Projection in the Drawing of the Human Figure*. Springfield, IL: Charles C. Thomas.
12. Buck, J.N. (1948). The house-tree-person techniques: A qualitative and quantitative scoring manual. *Journal of Clinical Psychology*, 4:151-159.
13. Oster, G.D. & Gould, P. (1987). *Using Drawings in Assessment and Therapy*. New York: Brunner/Mazel.
14. Urban, W.H. (1963). *The Draw-a-Person Catalog for Interpretive Analysis*. Los Angeles: Western Psychological Services.
15. Hemphill, B.J. (1982a). *The Evaluative Process in Psychiatric Occupational Therapy*. Thorofare, NJ: Slack.
16. Androes, L., Dreyfus, E.A., & Bloesch, M. (1965). Diagnostic test battery for occupational therapy. *American Journal of Occupational Therapy*, 19(2), 53-59.
17. Practice Division. (1988). *Mental Health Information Packet*. Rockville, MD: American Occupational Therapy Association.
18. Burns, R.C. & Kaufman, S.H. (1972). *Actions, Styles and Symbols in Kinetic Family Drawings (K-F-D)*. New York: Brunner/Mazel.
19. Siev, E. & Frieshtat, B. (1976). *Perceptual Dysfunction in the Adult Stroke Patient*. Thorofare, NJ: Charles B. Slack.
20. Hemphill, B.J. (1982b). *Training Manual for the BH Battery*. Thorofare, NJ: Slack.
21. Wald, J. (1983). Alzheimer's disease and the role of art therapy in its treatment. *American Journal of Art Therapy*, 22(2), 57-64.
22. Early, M.B. (1987). *Mental Health Concepts and Techniques for the Occupational Therapy Assistant*. New York: Raven Press.

23. Liebmann, M. (1986). *Art Therapy for Groups*. Cambridge, MA: Brookline Books.
24. Rhyne, J. (1973). *The Gestalt Art Experience*. Belmont, CA: Wadsworth Publishing Company, Inc.
25. Robbins, A. & Sibley, L.B. (1976). *Creative Art Therapy*. New York: Brunner/Mazel.
26. Department of the Army. (1971). *Craft Techniques in Occupational Therapy*. Washington DC: US Government Printing Office.
27. DiLeo, J.H. (1973). *Children's Drawings as Diagnostic Aids*. New York: Brunner/Mazel.
28. Gaitskell, C.D. & Hurwitz, A. (1975). *Children and Their Art*, 3rd ed. New York: Harcourt, Brace, Jovanovitch.
29. Drake, L.M. (September, 1988). Art media with aging adults: View from near the finish line. *Gerontology Special Interest Section Newsletter,* 11(3), 1-2.
30. Ogura, R. (1968). *The Lively Art of Ink Painting*. Tokyo: Japan Publications.

17
Other Frequently Used Crafts

▼

Introduction

Crafts become fads in a way similar to food and clothes. Photographs of occupational therapy in the 1920s and 1930s show basketry and working with straw.[1] Books of the 1940s and 1950s show pictures of woodworking and looms for weaving and knotting.[2-6] The books of the 1960s, have more adaptive equipment and industrial or vocational pictures.[7-9] By the 1970s, there were fewer craft photos, replaced by pictures of splints, pediatric developmental testing and adaptive equipment.[10-12] This trend continued into the 1980s, with more pictures of vocational and work-hardening activities.[13-15] Within each of these decades, there have been other crafts that have held the limelight in occupational therapy clinics for brief spans of time. New crafts continue to be developed that fit current treatment situations such as decreased hospital stays or increasing numbers of AIDS patients.

Frequency of Use

The term *minor media* is sometimes used to refer to crafts that receive less emphasis while they may still be useful activities.[16] The orientation of the person defining the category will decide which media will be defined as minor. In this text it means those crafts that are used less frequently, yet still have enough value to be something a therapist can use when necessary, even if they are not used often enough for the therapist to feel skilled in doing them. Crafts that could qualify as minor media are decoupage, stain frames, nature printing and silk screening. Each of these crafts will be discussed briefly.

Discussion of Individual Minor Media

Decoupage

This craft has a French name. *Couper*, the root word in decoupage, means *to cut* in that language. Some craft historians claim the craft developed in France and some say Italy. Decoupage was originally intended to be an inexpensive way of reproducing the look of oriental lacquer ware. Pictures were cut out and glued to lacquered objects, then covered with clear lacquer to simulate the handpainted designs on oriental furniture. It quickly spread to other countries as a decorative technique.

Though the original method took a great deal of time to complete, modern products have made it a simple and satisfying craft for patients. New one-coat finishes have been developed to simulate those that formerly required ten coats of varnish or lacquer.[17-19] Decoupage can be applied to glass, porcelain or wood. The techniques for wood are described below.

Supplies
- Wooden decoupage plaque;
- Fine sandpaper;
- Wood stain;
- Decoupage finish;
- Pictures from greeting cards or pictures printed on other thick paper;
- Scissors;
- Small glue brush;
- Finish brush with 2 1/2in. bristles;
- Cup to hold decoupage finish; and
- Brayer or rolling pin.

PROCESS
1. Sand wooden plaque.
2. Wipe on wood stain. Allow to dry.
3. Cut out picture and try it on plaque for correct placement.
4. If edges are thick, thin them by sanding edges gently from the back so they will be flat.
5. With small brush, apply decoupage finish, which works as glue, to the back of the picture.
6. Place the picture, glue side down, on the plaque.
7. With the rolling pin or brayer (Figure 17-1) gently roll out any bubbles under the picture. Allow this to dry.

8. Apply a coat of decoupage finish to the picture and wood and allow it to dry.

Perhaps the best thing about decoupage is that a very nice product can be produced so simply. It allows a patient with very diminished function to make a nice object. Most decoupage finish is neither flammable nor toxic so it is not a hazard for low-functioning patients. It can be used to preserve personally valuable mementos like graduation or birth announcements. The one drawback for the modern clinic is

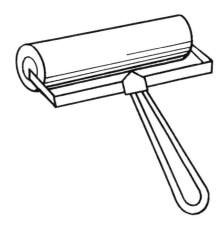

Figure 17-1
Brayer

the series of waiting periods while glue or finish dries. Though this craft is less used than it was in the 1970s, it is a traditional method that will continue to be useful.

Stain Frames

Stain frames are fairly new compared to other crafts in this text. It is a short-term structured process using preformed plastic (styrene) forms. Glass stain paints are applied to the areas between the raised outline ridges. The finished product simulates stained glass. They can be used as suncatchers or tree ornaments. Permanent markers or acrylic paints can be used for an opaque effect.

Stain frames are a simple one-step activity, simply applying the colors to the stain frame. Cleaning up and putting a hanger in the ring at top completes this project. Because of its simplicity it is well adapted to modern-day clinics where patients often have a time limited session and where patients are sicker at the time they are treated than they were in former times when hospital stays were longer. In some ways, stain frames are like paint-by-number in that the patient is not challenged by too many decisions.

Stain frames are appropriate for patients working on fine motor control. Because stain frames are unbreakable, they can be used with patients who have grip or balance problems and may tend to drop objects.

Nature Printing

This is another craft in which an extremely simple four-step process produces an interesting and clear design. Six inch by 9in. sun-sensitive paper with objects on it is exposed to the sun. Wherever the object blocks out the sun, the paper is white. Areas exposed to the sun become bright blue. The only materials needed are the nature print paper, objects for the design and tap water.

PROCESS

1. Arrange the objects on the paper. Possible objects could be keys, leaves, cut paper designs, buttons, lace or crochet doilies.
2. Put paper with objects in place in sun for 15 minutes.
3. Remove objects and immerse paper in tap water.
4. Spread wet paper on newspaper to dry. To keep wet paper from curling, tack each corner down to cardboard with straight pins.

Almost any patient will enjoy this rather magical craft process, however as a therapeutic media it is probably appropriate for patients who have poor attention spans and need quick gratification. Patients on sun-sensitive medication such as Thorazine and some antibiotics need to be cautioned about the hazards of staying out in the sun with their design. The nature print makes a nice design for the front of a greeting card or to decoupage.

Printing

The first printing was developed in China in approximately 200 AD. These first prints were what we call monoprints today, or simple prints. A design is made with ink and another paper is pressed on the ink to make a mirror image. Then it was discovered that stone carvings or seal rings could be used to print. The surface of the carving was rubbed with ink and then paper was pressed on the ink. A simple carved design could be used over and over. In about 600 AD, the Chinese discovered the process for woodblock printing in which a design was carved into a flat woodblock. The block was covered with ink by a brayer or roller (Figure 17-1) and then pressed onto the paper. The first European woodblock prints appeared in the 1400s. Metal etchings developed later in that same century. Lithography, printing with flat stones with an ink-absorbent design, was discovered in the late 1700s.

Silk screen on cloth, sometimes called serigraphy, was developed in the first decade of this century in England. This makes it a comparatively young craft. It is a more complex process of printing in which ink is pushed onto paper or cloth through a stencil design fixed on tightly stretched fine fabric mesh. T-shirts are commonly decorated this way. Its complexity may be the reason it is so little used.[20-22] Typesetting and printing presses have often been used in occupational therapy.[4,11,23-25] Printing presses are almost never found in clinics now. Few commercial establishments have typesetting any more. They use photo typesetting. The demise of the printing press in occupational therapy clinics parallels its demise in commercial print shops. Artists may be the main users of actual printing presses for the processes of etching an lithography.

Silk Screen

Silk screen designs can be blocked out by brushing glue, lacquer, lithographer's tushe or shellac right unto the screen. A lithographer's crayon can be used to draw on the cloth or a special silkscreen film can be affixed to the mesh. A simple way to achieve a silk screen effect is the paper stencil method. Materials needed for this process are:

- Silk screen box with mesh attached (Figure 17-2);
- Paper;
- Acrylic or water-soluble printer's ink;
- Squeegee; and
- Scissors;

PROCESS

1. Cover the work area with newspapers.
2. Place the paper on which the print will be made on the newspaper.
3. Cut a paper design and position it under the silk screen on top of the paper to be printed.
4. Squeeze ink unto the screen and use the squeegee to push the ink through cloth onto the design and the bottom paper. Do not thin the ink. Thicker ink produces a clearer design.
5. When the screen is lifted, the cut design will adhere to the silk. Remove the printed paper below and replace with a clean sheet.
6. Repeat steps four and five until desired number of prints are made.
7. Remove paper design and discard. Immediately wash screen and squeegee with soap and water.

This method produces only simple, one color designs. A thin paper used to make the cut design will result in a thin coat of ink on the printed paper. Thick paper used to make the design allows a thick layer of ink on the printed paper. Tracing paper or other nonabsorbent paper is not good for the cut design as it will not adhere to the mesh to allow

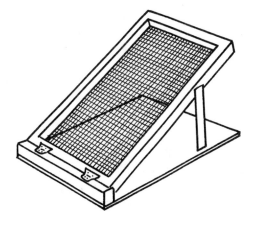

Figure 17-2
Silk Screen Frame

for more than one print. Physically this method requires good upper extremity strength and coordination, prehension and grasp.[21,26]

Linoleum Prints

The techniques for linoleum block and woodblock printing are basically the same. A design is cut into the top of the block, inked and printed. The picture is inverted in this printing process so all words or lettering must be carved backward.

Supplies

- Block with at least 1/8in. thick linoleum;
- Carbon paper;
- Linoleum lino cutters or wood carving tools;
- Brayer (Figure 17-1);
- 8in. x 11in. glass or lucite window pane;
- Water-soluble printer's ink
- 8 1/2in. x 11in. drawing paper or manila paper;
- Newspapers;
- Bracer board; and
- Paper towels.

PROCESS

1. Cover the work area with newspaper.
2. Reproduce the desired design on the linoleum surface using carbon paper.
3. Cut the outline of the design into the linoleum with a lino cutter, which has a small blade in a loop shape on the end of the handle.
4. Gouge out design where desired using a gouge with the block braced against a bracer board (Figure 6-10) for support and safety.
5. Run a proof on a paper towel
   a. Roll ink over glass pane with brayer.
   b. Roll inked brayer over linoleum surface.
   c. Press the linoleum onto the paper towel on a pad of newspapers
6. If the proof is acceptable, continue printing on the drawing paper.
7. If the proof is unacceptable, wash off the ink. Dry the block and continue carving out the linoleum and printing until a satisfactory proof is run.
8. Wash the block, brayer and inking pane with soap and water.[18,21]

Linoleum printing takes good upper extremity strength and control. Cutting the linoleum requires good hand strength and fine motor coordination. Use of the brayer elicits elbow flexion and extension. Some patients may substitute trunk motion for arm motion and should be observed and guided to achieve the movement desired.[26] Depressed or suicidal patients will require the usual precautions with sharp tools. Teenagers may enjoy these techniques but they are probably too difficult for children younger than eight or nine years of age.

Inner Tube Printing

This method of printing is similar to linoleum and woodblock printing during the actual printing process. However, the process of making the design to be printed is much easier. A design is drawn on a used tire inner tube. The design is cut out with regular craft scissors. The design pieces are arranged as desired on the woodblock background and glued in place with water-resistant glue. After the glue is dry, the linoleum printing process from step five onward is followed. Because this process uses fewer and less dangerous tools it can be used by children and lower-functioning patients. Because it is easier, it is also quicker and more adaptable for today's short hospital stays. All of these methods—wood, linoleum and inner tube block printing—produce attractive greeting cards and stationery.

Vegetable Prints

Vegetable prints make interesting repetitive designs for gift wrap, book covers or cloth.

Supplies

- Raw carrots, potatoes, turnips or other solid vegetables;
- Paring knife;
- Potato peeler;
- Ink stamp pad and ink;
- Paper towels;
- Paper or fabric to be printed; and
- Newspapers.

PROCESS

1. Cover work area with newspaper.
2. Cross-cut the vegetable so there is a flat surface for carving the design.
3. Trace a simple shaped design like a triangle, square, star or four-petal flower on the flat surface with the tip of the knife or a pen.
4. Incise the outline 1/4in. deep. This makes it easier to cut away or gouge out the background. The potato peeler may be useful for carving out corners of design.

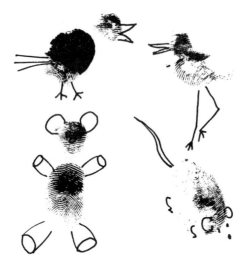

Figure 17-3
Fingerprint Designs

5. Press the cut surface on the inked stamp pad and print a proof on a paper towel.
6. If the proof is satisfactory, proceed to print the design on paper or cloth.
7. Clean up.

Because of the inexpensiveness and availability of the materials and tools, this is popular for all ages. The same upper extremity strength and coordination requirements and suicidal precautions of other printing apply to vegetable printing.

Fingerprint Design

Another kind of printing for all age groups is fingerprint designs. Simply press a finger or thumb on an inked stamp pad and press it on paper. When the print is dry, embellish it with arms, legs or other features to make an entertaining, easy design that requires almost no strength (Figure 17-3).

There are many other minor crafts that therapists can use to offer variety and richness to their activity choices in working with patients. Craft materials manufacturers continue to develop new ideas for projects to make in the clinic. A visit to craft vendor booths at conferences is an opportunity to learn about these new materials and projects.

References

1. Howe, M. & Schwartzberg, S. (1986). *A Functional Approach to Group Work in Occupational Therapy.* Philadelphia: Lippincott.
2. Colson, J.H.C. (1944). *The Rehabilitation of the Injured: Occupational Therapy.* London: Cassell and Company.
3. Department of the Army. (1951). *Occupational Therapy.* Washington DC: US Government Printing Office.
4. Dunton, W.R. & Licht, S. (1957). *Occupational Therapy Principles and Practice.* Springfield, IL: Charles C. Thomas.
5. Haworth, N.A. & Macdonald, E.M. (1946). *Theory of Occupational Therapy.* Baltimore: Williams & Wilkins.
6. Willard, H.S. & Spackman, C.S. (1947). *Principles of Occupational Therapy.* Philadelphia: Lippincott.
7. Jones, M.S. (1960). *An Approach to Occupational Therapy.* London: Butterworth.
8. MacDonald, E.M. (Ed.). (1960a). *Occupational Therapy in Rehabilitation.* Baltimore: Williams & Wilkins.
9. MacDonald, E.M. (Ed.) (1960b). *Occupational Therapy in Rehabilitation.* Baltimore: Williams and Wilkins.

10. Jones, M.S. (1977). *An Approach to Occupational Therapy.* London: Butterworth.

11. Hopkins, H.L. & Smith, H.D. (1978). *Willard and Spackman's Occupational Therapy,* 5th ed. Philadelphia: Lippincott.

12. Willard, H.S. & Spackman, C.E. (1971). *Occupational Therapy,* 4th ed. Philadelphia: Lippincott.

13. Hopkins, H.L. & Smith, H.D. (1983). *Willard and Spackman's Occupational Therapy,* 6th ed. Philadelphia: Lippincott.

14. Hopkins, H.L. & Smith, H.D. (1988). *Willard and Spackman's Occupational Therapy,* 7th ed. Philadelphia: Lippincott.

15. Ryan, S. (Ed.). (1986). *The Certified Occupational Therapy Assistant: Roles and Responsibilities.* Thorofare, NJ: Slack.

16. Wilkinson, V.C. & Heater, S.L. (1979). *Therapeutic Media and Techniques of Application: A Guide for Activities Therapists.* New York: Van Nostrand Reinhold Company.

17. Bodger, L. & Brock, D. (1976). *The Crafts Engagement Calendar 1976.* New York: Universe Books.

18. Reader's Digest. (1979). *Crafts and Hobbies.* Pleasantville, NY: The Reader's Digest Association Inc.

19. VanZandt, E. (1973). *Crafts for Fun and Profit.* London: Aldus Books.

20. Hobson, J. (1970). *Dyed and Printed Fabrics.* Wood Ridge, NJ: The Dryad Press.

21. Kent, C. & Cooper, M. (1966). *Simple Printmaking.* New York: Watson-Gauptill Publications.

22. Reader's Digest. (1979). *Crafts and Hobbies.* Pleasantville, NY: The Reader's Digest Association Inc.

23. Department of the Army. (1951). *Occupational Therapy.* Washington, DC: US Government Printing Office.

24. Department of the Army. (1971). *Craft Techniques in Occupational Therapy.* Washington DC: US Government Printing Office.

25. Office of the Surgeon General. (1945). *Curing by Printing: Printing Activities in Occupational Therapy.* New York: American Type Founders.

26. Hamill, C.M. & Oliver, R.C. (1989). *Therapeutic Activity for the Handicapped Elderly.* Gaithersburg, MD: Aspen Publishers.

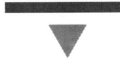

18
Miscellaneous Creative Media

Introduction

While we usually do not think of performance activities as craft, it is common in theater work to speak of the acting craft. A craft is also defined as an activity that is done skillfully and ingeniously.[1] This definition is used in this chapter to explain inclusion of face painting, clowning, pantomime and magic. Face painting, clowning and mime, each an individual craft with its own merit, do fit together. Faces are painted before both clowning and miming. Clowns wear make-up and also include pantomime in their acts. Most pantomime artists paint their faces and appear clownish. The three are often an integral part of a whole act. Noncompetitive games are also mentioned here as creative treatment media.

Face Painting

This creative medium, face painting, is often done at craft fairs and festivals where clowns and mime artists are also seen. Make-up for actors and clowns has been around for centuries. Face painting is a direct descendent of clown make-up and can be done with cosmetic face make-up. However, it is more permanent and gives a professional look if done with grease paint or theatrical make-up. Cosmetic make-up is more likely to run and smear. Grease paint will last longer and tolerate more wear and tear.

Supplies

- Paper and pencil;
- Grease paint;
- Make-up brushes;
- Baby oil;
- Talcum powder; and
- Facial tissue.

PROCESS

1. It is best to draw a face with a plan for the make-up first (Figure 18-1).
2. Brushes are used for applying face paint or grease paint. Apply colors in this order, white, pastels, primary colors and, last, black.
3. Powder each color after applying it. Brush excess powder away with a powder brush.
4. Clean grease paint from brushes with baby oil. Wipe brushes dry.

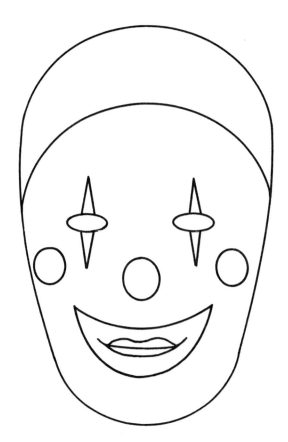

Figure 18-1
Make-Up Face Plan

5. Disinfect brushes between patients.
6. Check face paint in the mirror.

The main precautions for using face paint are to be aware of allergies to make-up and to avoid breathing the talcum powder. Face painting should be avoided by respiratory patients or those with dermatitis or acne.

Children and teenagers especially enjoy face painting. Face painting is almost a prerequisite for clowning and mime. In both of these crafts most of the face is usually painted. Often, for children and teens, just a flower, teardrop or leaf design is sufficient rather than painting the whole face.[2-5]

Clowning

Almost every culture has some form of clown character. Clowning is a kind of acting in which the actor wears stylized make-up and a costume. There is a cartoonlike quality to a clown act. Clowns help us laugh at our own human foibles and inadequacies. Clowning offers patients the opportunity to act silly in an acceptable caricature of themselves or others.[4-6]

Clowning takes thought and planning, which are areas of frequent therapeutic focus in cognition and goal setting. Patients must think through the effect they wish to achieve, then plan how they can accomplish that effect. There are opportunities to work in pairs or groups as most clown acts involve team work. Generally, the patient will have to be functioning well enough to appreciate humorous situations. The severely depressed, schizophrenic and mentally retarded patients may have difficulty organizing and carrying out comedy scenarios, while they may enjoy watching others do clowning. Some patients with personality disorders could use this medium to exaggerate their aberrant responses to situations and people. Imagine a borderline personality-disordered patient clutching at someone and screeching "Don't leave me alone. I can't stand it." Alcoholics and drug abusers may enjoy playing the drunk. This process can help them develop insight into society's reaction to them.

For the physically disabled, playing the comical side of disability can offer an emotional outlet for feelings about their situation. There has been an effort to use comedy to increase public awareness of disabilities. Comedy and clowning are seen as ways to alter the public's attitude about this sensitive subject.[7]

Mime

Mime and pantomime are used interchangeably here, as one term is just an abbreviation of the other. Gesture and pose, which are the bases of pantomime, were probably the first human means of communication. They are the most universal forms of communication. When communicating with someone who speaks a foreign language, we liberally augment speech with gestures.

Pantomime means basically storytelling through bodily movements and facial expression. Its origins are often attributed to the Greeks who so richly developed drama and its associated techniques such as mime. Tribal dances of Native Americans, Arabs and Africans are indeed pantomime dances. They often do a pantomime of the hunt as preparation for actually going to hunt. Most European and British people have developed forms of pantomime. Charlie Chaplin may be the best mime artist America produced. Acting is native to humans and comes before speaking in the same way drawing comes before writing.[1,8,9]

The main purpose in using mime with patients is to help them learn to communicate better and understand the body language of others. Second, pantomime is for fun. Third, it may be used to enact or reenact a patient's problem situation. Start each mime session with a warm-up. In warming up, the patients can stretch, explore their body movements by keeping all but one part fixed, or by anchoring one part and moving all the others. Music or rhythm instruments can be used to stimulate movement. An appropriate warm-up for children ages three to eight years could be pretending to be a wind-up toy. The therapist would demonstrate with a real wind-up toy, then pretend to wind the child up. Other warm-ups for children could be pantomimes of different kinds of balls, animals or vehicles. Warm-ups for children ages eight to 12 years could be occupational or sports related such as shooting a basketball. Teenagers may relate more to romantic dramatization or putting on make-up and clothes for warm-ups. This allows patients to get into the mood. Adults can be asked to do movements that simulate openness or closedness, nearness or distance. Such options allow adult patients to use just a hand if they are inhibited about body movement or to use the whole body if they feel less self-conscious. Older adults may enjoy pantomiming famous people like Franklin Delano Roosevelt and his famous cigarette holder, the expressionless look of Jack Benny or the come hither look of Hedy Lamar.

The next step would be to have patients suggest scenarios for mime. Some groups of patients may need prompting before developing a list of possible scenarios. Alcoholics may play a bartender refusing to sell a drunk another drink. Hospitalized patients may mime complaining to the dietitian about their food or to the orthotist about their appliance. Almost any concrete or intrapsychic problem can be mimed if patients think through exactly the message they wish to communicate. By paying attention to the details of communication, patients are often able to learn how they affect other people. Scenes can be replayed until the patient or audience feels satisfied with the pantomime. In closing a mime session, patients may enact the various goodbye rituals we use—waving, hugging or shaking hands.[8,10-17] Most clinics will not have the time to put on stage makeup—face painting for a mime session, however, if a group begins to elaborate its ideas and plan a performance, this may be an occasion to experiment with make-up or grease paint.

Magic

Occupational therapists have been using magic as a medium of treatment for the last half decade. Magic in many cases means the supernatural, casting a spell or dark scary things we don't understand. For occupational therapy it is not supernatural or scary. It is a novelty for patients who have become bored with other types of treatment such as repetitive exercise. Project Magic works to link therapists and magicians in order to facilitate their working together in teaching magic tricks to patients. They provide a trick book along with lists of local magicians who have an interest in working with patients. Tricks are used with one-handed patients, head trauma patients or any patients who need to improve manual dexterity.[18] There are a good number of books on magic to be found in the juvenile section of the library.[19-23] Tricks run the gamut from, for example, the *magic penny*, in which the fledgling magician uses words to trick by saying "I bet if I put down my penny you won't be able to jump over it" and then puts the penny down on top of the other person's head or shoulder[20] to sophisticated card tricks. All tricks require practice to be performed smoothly.[19] Practice of difficult processes and movements are integral to patient improvement of coordination, control, sequencing and cognition.

Noncompetitive Games

As we have come to realize that cooperation compared to competition produces better performance outcomes, there has been a trend toward developing and using cooperative activities.[24,25] In the 1970s, as the words *a happening* came to describe a group of people enjoying themselves together, occupational therapists began to use some these happening activities with patients. Parachute games and "Knots" are two that are commonly used with many different kinds of patients.[26,27] Other cooperative game books soon followed for both children and adults.[28,29] The basic idea for all these activities is that people should be able to play together with each other, not against each other. When human energy is used against another, often someone gets hurt physically or psychologically. As the New Games Foundation motto asserts "Play Hard, Play Fair, Nobody Hurt."[28]

Some noncompetitive board games have also been used by occupational therapists for more than a decade. One such game is *The Ungame*. It is a values clarification game with decks of question cards, markers and board positions.

Originally it had one model intended for all groups. Later, special decks of question cards were developed for children, all ages, and so forth.[30] It is the experience of the author that almost any diagnostic patient group will enjoy The Ungame. *Slice of Life* is another board game for improving communication, self-image, leisure use and time management.[31] For alcohol and drug abusers, *Sobriety* is a board game asking the hard questions about staying sober after discharge. For each of these games, literacy is almost a necessity. A therapist can adapt the rules so one person does all the reading to avoid putting an illiterate player on the spot. Each of these games is noncompetitive.

An important point for the student of activities for occupational therapy is that there are new, exciting ideas for therapy being developed constantly. Because of the wide spectrum of available treatments, occupational therapists have a great deal of freedom in matching their patient with appropriate activities.

References

1. *Webster's Seventh New Collegiate Dictionary.* (1969). Springfield, MA: G & C Merriam Company.
2. Baygan, L. (1982). *Make-up for the Theater, Film and Television.* New York: Drama Book Publishers.
3. Buchman, L.G. (1975). *Stage Makeup.* New York: Watson-Guptill Publications.
4. Harris, S.M. (1985). *This is My Trunk.* New York: Atheneum.
5. Stolzenberg, M. (1981). *Clown for Circus and Stage.* New York: Sterling Publishing Co.
6. Harzberg, H. & Moss, A. (1924). *Slapstick and Dumbbell.* New York: Joseph Lawren.
7. Milner, M. (1987a). Actors avoid preaching to show lighter side of living with disability. *OT Week,* 1(42), 12-14.
8. Keysell, P. (1975). *Mime: Themes and Motifs.* Boston: Plays, Inc., Publishers.
9. Pardoe, T.E. (1931). *Pantomimes for Stage and Study.* New York: Benjamin Blom.
10. Alberts, D. (1971). *Pantomime: Elements and Exercises.* Lawrence, KS: The University of Kansas Press.
11. Aubert, C. (1976). *The Art of Pantomime.* New York: Arno Press.
12. Blatner, H.A. (1973). *Acting In: Practical Applications of Psychodramatic Methods.* New York: Springer Publishing.
13. Buchan, L.G. (1972). *Roleplaying and the Educable Mentally Retarded.* Belmont, CA: Fearon Publishers.
14. Corsini, R.J. & Cardone, S. (1966). *Roleplaying in Psychotherapy.* Chicago: Aldine Publishing Company.
15. Gray, V. & Percival, R.. (1962). *Music, Movement and Mime for Children.* Toronto: Oxford.
16. Weisberg, N. & Wilder, R. (1985). *Creative Arts With Older Adults: A Sourcebook.* New York: Human Sciences Press.
17. Wethered, A.G. (1973). *Movement and Drama in Therapy.* Boston, MA: Boston Plays, Inc.
18. Milner, M. (1987b). Occupational therapist and entertainer put magic into rehabilitation program. *OT Week,* 1(50): 12-13.
19. Gibson, W. (1980). *Big Book of Magic for All Ages.* Garden City, NY: Doubleday and Company.
20. Lopshire, R. (1969). *It's Magic?* New York: MacMillan Publishing.
21. Severn, B. (1964). *Magic in Your Pockets.* New York: David McKay Company.

22. Severn, B. (1965). *Magic Shows You Can Give*. New York: David McKay Company.
23. Severn, B. (1977). *Magic With Coins and Bills*. New York: David McKay Company.
24. Kohn, A. (1986). *No Contest*. New York: Houghton Mifflin.
25. Rabow, G. (1988). The cooperative edge. *Psychology Today*, 22(1), 54-58.
26. Fluegelman, A. (Ed.). (1976). *The New Games Book*. Tiburon, CA: Headlands Press.
27. French, R., Horvat, M., & Alexander, F. (1983). *Parachute Movement Activities—A Complete Parachute Movement Program for Elementary School and Beyond*. Byron, CA: Front Row Discovery.
28. Fluegelman, A. (Ed.). (1981). *More New Games!* Tiburon, CA: Headlands Press.
29. Orlich, T. (1978). *The Cooperative Sports and Games Book: Challenge Without Competition*. New York: Pantheon Books.
30. Zakich, R. (1983). *The Ungame Company*. Anaheim, CA.
31. Michelson, B. (1985). *A Slice of Life*. 330 Sycamore Road, DeKalb, Illinois 60115.

Appendices

Appendix I

Vendors of Materials Described in this Text

AMACO
American Art Clay Co., Inc.
4717 W. 16th Street
Indianapolis, Indiana 46222
1-317-244-6871

Attainment Co. (Instructional curricula
    for food preparation)
P.O. Box 103
Oregon, Wisconsin 53575
1-800-327-4269

Career Aids (Instructional curricula for
food preparation)
20417 Nordhoff Street, Dept. AH7
Chatsworth, California 91311
1-818-341-2535

Computer Solutions
P.O. Box 658
Danville, Virginia 24543-0658
1-804-793-0181

Computer Support Corporation
15926 Midway Road
Dallas, Texas 75244
1-214-661-8960

Creative Crafts International
16 Plains Road
P.O. Box 819
Essex, Connecticut 06426
1-203-767-2101

Dick Blick (Art supplies)
P.O. Box 1267
Galesburg, Illinois 61401

Fred Sammons, Inc.
    (Adaptive equipment)
Box 32
Brookfield, Illinois 60513-0032
1-800-323-5547

Glimakra Looms 'n Yarn Inc.
1304 Scott Street
Petaluma, California 94952
1-707-762-3362

Intuit Computing
1915 Huguenot Road
Richmond, Virginia 23235
1-800-633-1221

Mid-South Ceramic Supply Co.
1230 4th Avenue North
Nashville, Tennessee 37280
1-615-242-0300

Midwest Clay Co.
8001 Grand Avenue South
Bloomington, Minnesota 55420
1-800-328-9380

Nasco Arts and Crafts
1524 Princeton Avenue
Modesto, California 95352
1-209-529-6957

Nasco Arts and Crafts
901 Janesville Avenue
Fort Atkinson, Wisconsin 53538
1-800-558-9595

Polarware Software (Computers)
1055 Paramount Parkway
Batavia, Illinois 60510
1-312-232-1984

Queue Inc. (Instructional curricula for
   food preparation)
562 Boston Avenue
Bridgeport, Connecticut 06610
1-800-232-2224

Robert J. Golka Co. (Leathercraft)
400 Warren Avenue
P.O. Box 676
Brockton, Massachusetts 02403
1-508-586-7320

Royal Arts and Crafts
650 Ethel Street N.W.
P.O. Box 93486
Atlanta, Georgia
1-404-876-6428

S & S Arts and Crafts
Colchester, Connecticut 06415
1-203-537-3451

Sax Arts & Crafts
P.O. Box 2002
Milwaukee, Wisconsin 53201
1-800-558-6696

Slice of Life, A
330 Sycamore Road
DeKalb, Illinois 60115
1-815-756-1140 or 1-815-756-1521
ext. 3363

Smith & Nephew Roylan, Inc. (Adapative
   equipment)
N93 W14475 Whittaker Way
Menomonee Falls, Wisconsin 53051
1-800-558-8633

Sobriety
P.O. Box 6630
Reno, Nevada 89513-6630

Tandy Leather Company
P.O. Box 2934
Fort Worth, Texas 76113
Look in telephone book for local Tandy
   Store number.

Triarco Arts & Crafts
14650 28th Avenue North
Plymouth, Minnesota 55447
1-800-328-3360

Ungame Company, The
Anaheim, California 92806

Vanguard Crafts, Inc.
P.O. Box 340170
Brooklyn, New York 11234
1-718-337-5188

Victorian Video Productions
Handicraft Videos
1304 Scott Street
Petaluma, California 94952
1-707-762-3362

Appendix II

▼

Annotated Bibliography

This appendix presents an annotated bibliography for the craft areas mentioned in this book. These references are different from the ones used in the text. Some are for the craftsperson who wishes for more advanced techniques while others are a more thorough presentation of crafts described herein and some are historical accounts of the craft's development. There is also a listing for specific cultural crafts and one for other books on crafts for the clinic and for the handicapped.

Woodworking
Woodcraft
by Bernard S. Mason
Cranbury, New Jersey: A.S. Barnes and Co., Inc., 1973.
Crafts for living in the woods, bark crafts, Indian and American pioneer woodcrafts, tools and games.

Arts and Crafts Objects Children Can Make for the Home
by Jean Lyon
West Nyack, New York: Parker Publishing Company, Inc., 1976.
A chapter on woodcraft techniques with lumber scraps for children.

The Complete Handbook of Power Tools
by George R. Drake
Reston, Virginia: Reston Publishing Company, Inc., 1975.
A complete presentation with photographs of most power tools, including precautions, used by occupational therapists.

Amateur Craftman's Cyclopedia
by Popular Science Monthly
New York: Popular Science Publishing Company, Inc., 1937.
While most of this old how-to-do-it book is on woodcrafts, there are sections on electricity, radio, metal craft, photograph and weather measurement tools.

Wood Carving and Whittling
by Popular Science Monthly
New York: Popular Science Publishing
Company, Inc., 1936.
Thorough instructions for all kinds of
carving.

Woodworking
by Willis H. Wagner
South Holland, Illinois: The Goodheart—
Willcox Co., Inc., 1975.
A basic text presenting power and hand
tools. Shows how to do many small wood
projects.

Easy Ways to Expert Woodworking
by Robert Scharff
New York: McGraw Hill Book Company,
Inc., 1956.
Describes and has photos of most power
shop tools and processes. Does not deal
with hand tools. No project designs or
plans.

Bench Woodwork
by John L. Feirer
Peoria, Illinios: C.A. Bennett Co., 1972.
Emphasis on hand tools though power
tools are also presented. Plans for many
projects are in the back.

Leathercraft
Leathercraft
by Fred W. Zimmerman
South Holland, Illinois: The Goodheart-
Wilcox Co., Inc., 1969.
A basic book with traditional projects,
designs, tools and techniques.

Creative Leathercraft
by Grete Peterson
New York: Sterling Publishing Co., Inc.,
1960.
A simple, small, well-illustrated book
with many traditional projects but also
leather embroidery and leather mosaic.

Leather Work Including Glove Making
by Albert H. Crampton
London, Frederick Warne & Co., Ltd.,
1930.
An abbreviated description of tools and
processes. It has a section on leather
applique.

Modern Leather Design
by Don Willcox
New York: Watson-Guptill Publications,
1969.
Presents process from raw hide to
finished leather. Thorough presentation
of tools, lacing and tooling processes.
Modern artistic designs for clothing,
jewelry, furniture and art.

Leathercraft
by Chris H. Groneman
Peoria, Illinois: Charles A. Bennett Co.,
Inc., 1963.
A basic book with traditional small
projects.

Needlework
*Arts and Crafts Objects Children Can
Make for the Home*
by Jean Lyon
West Nyack, New York: Parker
Publishing Company, Inc., 1976.
A chapter on stitchery projects for both
girls and boys.

Crafts for the Classroom
by Earl W. and Marlene M. Linderman
New York: MacMillan Publishing Co.,
Inc., 1977.
Easy-to-follow directions for many
projects with children.

Design in Fabric and Thread
by Aileen Murray
London: Watson-Guptill Publications,
1969.
Innovative designs for clothing,
wallhangings and other decorations.
Many photographs in both color and
black and white.

Classics for Needlepoint
by Susan Witt
Birmingham, Alabama: Oxmoor House,
1981.
Basic stitches, decorative stitches,
bargello and basketweave. Contains
many designs and patterns.

120 Needlepoint Design Projects
by Barnes and David Blake
New York: Crown Publishers, Inc., 1974.
From kinds of canvas to dozens of
designs.

Needlepoint Book
by Sylvia Sidney
New York: Van Nostrand Reinhold
Company, 1968.
Contains an index of stitches and how to
transfer designs.

Quilting as a Hobby
by Dorothy Brightbill
New York: Sterling Publishing Co., Inc.,
1964.
A brief history. Describes trapunto,
applique and traditional American
designs.

*Quilting, Patchwork, Applique and
Trapunto*
by Thelma R. Newman
New York: Crown Publishers, Inc., 1974.
A book to stimulate artists. Photographs
of historical and traditional works.

Knitting Without Tears
by Elizabeth Zimmerman
New York: Charles Scribrer's Sons, 1971.
From basic stitches to washing the
sweater. Not enough pictures for
beginners.

The Big Book of Knitting
by Isabelle Stevenson
New York: The Greystone Press, 1948.
Good diagrams and photos. Dozens of
projects. Some complex decorative
techniques.

Knitting Made Easy
by Barbara Aytes
Garden City, New York: Doubleday and
Company, Inc., 1970.
Photographs are not easy to understand.
For the advanced knitter no matter what
the title says.

Copper and Metal
Living Crafts
by George Bernard Hughes
Freeport, New York: Books for Libraries
Press, 1954.
Has four chapters on various metal
crafts. Contains history as well as
descriptions of 14 other crafts.

*Arts and Crafts Objects Children Can
Make for the Home*
by Jean Lyon
West Nyack, New York: Parker
Publishing Company, Inc., 1976.
Has a chapter on simple metal projects
for children.

Metal Projects
by John R. Walker
South Holland, Illinois: The Goodheart-
Wilcox Co., Inc., 1966.
Bending, welding, soldering and riveting
over 50 projects.

Coppercraft and Silver Made at Home
by Karl Robert Kramer and Nora Kramer
Philadelphia: Chilton Company Book
Division, 1957.
Thorough presentation of cutting,
shaping and riveting metal. Shows many
possible projects.

Fun With Colored Foil
by Manfred Burggraf
New York: Watson-Guptill Publications,
1969.
Good illustrations for cutting and
shaping many decorative small projects.

Mosaics
Modern Mosaic Techniques
by Janice Lovoos and Felice Paramore
New York: Watson-Guptill Publications,
1967.
For the artist. Wonderful photographs.

The Art of Making Mosaics
by Louisa Jenkins and Barbara Mills
Princeton, New Jersey: D. Van Nostrand
Company, Inc., 1957.
Discusses materials. Has a chapter on
children's mosaics and church art.

Mosaic Making
by Helen Hutton
New York: Reinhold Publishing
Corporation, 1966.
Step-by-step presentation of various
projects. How to
make, glaze and fire your own mosaic
tiles.

Mosaics: Principles and Practice
by Joseph L. Young
New York: Reinhold Publishing
Corporation, 1963.
Has some history. Many large mural-size
projects.

Course in Making Mosaics
by Joseph L. Young
New York: Reinhold Publishing
Corporation, 1956.
Lots of history. All black and white
pictures.

Ceramics
Crafts for the Classroom
by Earl W. and Marlene M. Lindermann
New York: MacMillan Publishing Co.,
Inc., 1977.
Simple clay and sculpture for the
classroom.

Glazes for the Potter
by William Ruscoe
New York: St. Martin's Press, 1974.
History of glazes. Complicated chemical
formulas. Not for the beginner.

Making Pottery Without a Wheel
by F. Carlton Ball and Janice Lovoos
New York: Van Nostrand Reinhold
Company, 1965.
Simple techniques and wonderful
textures with simple household items.

Fundamentals of Hobby Ceramics
by Bill Thompson
Livonia, Michigan: Scott Advertising and
Publishing Co., 1975.
On pouring molds and numerous surface
decoration techniques, some quite
complex.

Introducing Handbuilt Pottery
by Tony Volly
New York: Watson-Guptill Publications,
1973.
Good photographs of simple and complex
construction and decoration techniques.
Artistic works.

The Self-Reliant Potter
by Andrew Holden
New York: Van Nostrand Reinhold
Company, 1984.
For the rugged individualist who likes to
make everything from scratch. A plan for
how to get many materials almost free in
your own community.

Ceramics Techniques & Projects
by Elizabeth Hogan, supervising editor
Menlo Park, California: Lane Magazine
& Book Company, 1973.
Basic techniques for the hobby potter.
Hand-building and wheel, no molds.
Paper cover.

Pottery Designs
by David Close
London: B. T. Batsford, Ltd., 1984.
Photos and description of five basic
techniques: slipware, pinch pots, slabs,
modeling and press molds.

Step-By-Step Ceramics
by Jolyen Hofsted
New York: Golden Press, 1967.
A well-illustrated introduction to basic
principles and techniques. Photographs
of stimulating designs. Paper cover.

Weaving, Latchook, Macramé, Fibers
*Arts and Crafts Objects Children Can
Make for the Home*
by Jean Lyon
West Nyack, New York: Parker
Publishing Company Inc., 1976.
Has a chapter on simple weaving for
children.

Crafts for the Classroom
by Earl W. and Marlene M. Lindermann
New York: MacMillan Publishing Co.,
Inc., 1977.
Thorough presentation of terms with
simple directions for weaving and
macramé.

Elements of Weaving
by Azalea Stuart Thorpe and Jack Lenor
Larsen
Garden City, New York: Doubleday and
Company, Inc., 1967.
Has history. Concentration on four-
harness weaving.

Introducing Weaving
by Phyl Shillinglaw
New York: Watson-Guptill Publications, 1972.
Mostly simple looms. Presents dyes and various fibers.

Weaving Without a Loom
by Sarita R. Rainey
Worchester, Massachusetts: Davis Publications, Inc., 1972.
Includes God's Eyes, paper, latchook, card weaving and more. Pictures of artistic creations.

Weaving for Amateurs
by Helen Coates
London: The Studio Publications, 1946.
From small table loom, to four-harness loom, to dying, carding and spinning.

Macramé and Other Projects for Knitting Without Needles
by Peggy Boehm
New York: Gramercy Publishing Company, 1963.
Ideas for many projects but diagrams are fuzzy.

Ojos de Dios: Eye of God
by Charles Albaum
New York: Grosset and Dunlap, 1972.
From the basics to complex tribal designs with illustrations and photographs.

Macramé
by Ann Stearns
New York: Arco Publishing Company, Inc., 1975.
Elaborate belts, jewelry and clothes.

Fun With String
by Joseph Leeming
New York: Frederick A. Stokes Company, 1940.
Tricks and games, knots, macramé, braiding, handweaving, card weaving, spool knitting. Good diagrams.

Paper Crafts
Arts and Crafts Objects Children Can Make for the Home
by Jean Lyon
West Nyack, New York: Parker Publishing Company Inc., 1976.
Has a chapter on simple paper projects for children.

Crafts for the Classroom
by Earl W. and Marlene M. Linderman
New York: MacMillan Publishing Co., Inc., 1977.
Discusses developmental skills for art with children. Has many paper projects for children.

Modern Origami
by James Minoru Sakoda
New York: Simon and Schuster, 1969.
A nice progression from basic to complex origami.

Creative Origami
by Kunihiko Kasahara
London: Sir Issac Pitman and Son, Ltd., 1970.
Clear diagrams and photos of traditional forms as well as new artistic creations. One hundred different designs.

Art in Paper
by Carson I.A. Ritchie
South Brunswick: A.S. Barnes, 1976.
Silhouettes, decoupage, collage, paper sculpture, oriental cut paper. A short history on each one.

The Paper Book 187 Things to Make
by Don Munson and Allianora Rosse
New York: Charles Scribner's Sons, 1970.
Greeting cards, holiday decorations, dolls, costumes, buildings, animals. Good diagrams and directions.

Paper Sculpture
by Tadeusz Lipski
London: The Studio, Ltd., 1947.
A small book. Simple to complex. Ten projects.

Paper Folding and Paper Sculpture
by Kenneth Ody
Buchanan, New York: Emerson Books, Inc., 1976.
A wide variety of uses of cutting, scoring and folding. Good diagrams.

Creating With Corrugated Paper
by Rolf Hartung
New York: Reinhold Publishing, 1966.
Interesting designs, a maze, dolls, animals, vehicles, all from corrugated paper.

Paper People
by Michael Grater
New York: Taplinger Publishing
Company, 1970.
Many toys, puppets, dolls and novelties.
Some period people.

Cooking

Creative Food Experiences for Children
by Mary T. Goodwin and Gerry Pollen
Washington DC: Center for Science in the
Public Interest, 1974.
An easy-to-use format in this
comprehensive cookbook for children
though the print is too small for children.
Has nutrition information and ethnic
foods.

*Kitchen Classroom: Learning Through
Cooking*
by Shannon Wall-Mangum and Robin
Franklin Matthew
Covington, Louisiana: M and M
Therapeutics, 1990.
This cooking curriculum by two
occupational therapists has activities for
teaching concepts related to cooking, food
and feelings about eating. Some
worksheets can be copied for use.

Drawing and Painting

Anyone Can Paint Pictures
by Alfred Paddy Kerr
New York: Pitman Publishing
Corporation, 1960.
Simplified instructions for oil and
watercolor painting. Most illustrations
and pictures in black and white.

*The Artist's Handbook of Materials and
Techniques*
by Richard Mayer
New York: The Viking Press, 1948.
Comprehensive for technical problems.
Oils, tempera, watercolor, pastel crayons,
pigment compositions, chemistry and
murals.

*The Artist's Handbook of Materials and
Techniques*
by Ralph Mayer (Rev. ed.)
New York: The Viking Press, 1957.
A classic manual for the studio artist.
Comprehensive.

Weekend Painter
by Lawrence V. Burton
New York: Whittlesey House, 1948.
From basic color mixing to how to take
criticism.

Oil Painting for the Beginner
by Frederic Taukes (3rd ed.)
New York: Watson-Guptill Publications,
1965.
Large print. Color perspective, portraits,
landscapes.

*The Creative Way to Draw Heads and
Portraits*
by Authur Zaidenberg
New York: Cornerstone Library, 1969.
A step-by-step progression from simple
lines, anatomy, separate facial features,
shading and special problems.

The Joy of Painting
by Arthur Zaidenberg
Garden City, New York: Hanover House,
1955.
Mostly human figure drawing and
painting.

Introduction to the Visual Arts
edited by S. Ralph Maurello
New York: Tudor Publishing Company,
1968.
A basic description of art materials and a
thorough, step-by-step course in the
elements of drawing, color theory,
perspective, decorative design and other
fundamentals of art. Well-illustrated
with both color and black and white.

Painting for Children
by Lois Thomasson Horne
New York: Reinhold Book Corporation,
1968.
Gives basic materials, equipment and
techniques commonly used by teachers of
children. Examples of paintings by age
categories from 5 to 12 years old.

*Finger Tip Magic: Theory and Practice in
the Art of Finger Painting*
by Margaret O'Brien
Springfield, Massachusetts: Milton
Bradley Company, 1948.
An 18-page brochure with demonstration
pictures of different techniques and
effects.

Creating With Crayon
by Lothar Kampmann
New York: Reinhold Beck Corporation,
1967.
Techniques for using wax crayons.
Wonderful color illustrations and
examples of children's work. Good index.

Printing
Elementary Screen Printing
by Albert Kosloff
Chicago, Illinois: Naz-dar Company,
1972.
A small book with a few illustrations.
Describes photographic process.

Screen Printing Process
by Albert Kosloff
Cincinnati, Ohio: The Signs of The Times
Publishing Company, 1964.
A well-illustrated book with both
commercial and studio
printing described.

*The Complete Book of Silk Screen
Printing Production*
by J.J. Biegeleisen
New York: Dover Publications, Inc., 1963.
Thorough with history, techniques,
products, for artist and commercial
production.

The Art of the Print
by Fritz Eichenberg
New York: Harry N. Abrams, Inc.,
Publishers, 1976.
Reproduction of many masterpieces,
history of all techniques, lengthy
description of techniques.

Twentieth Century Graphics
by Jean Adhemar
New York: Praeger Publishers, 1971.
Mostly history. Little on how to do
techniques.

The Art of Etching
by E.S. Lumsden
New York: Dover Publications, Inc., 1962.
A history and how-to-do-it book of
drypoint etching, soft-ground etching and
aquatint. Thorough step-by-step
presentation with illustrations.

Ethnic or Culture
Southwestern Arts and Crafts
by Nancy Krenz and Patricia Byrnes
Santa Fe, New Mexico: The Sunstone
Press, 1979.
Contains Mexican and Indian Crafts,
recipes, music and dance for
kindergarten through 6th grade.

The Craftsman in America
by the National Geographic Society
Washington, DC: Special Publications
Division, 1975.
Historic as well as modern crafts
developed in America. Not a how-to-do-it
book.

African Crafts and Craftsmen
by René Gardi
New York: Van Nostrand Reinhold
Company, 1969.
Large print and wonderful photographs
of a variety of crafts from raw materials to
finished product from across that
continent.

West African Weaving
by Venice Lamb
London: Gerald Duckworth and Co., Ltd.,
1975.
Tribal maps show origins of various
weaves. Many photos of weavers at work.

Other Craft Books for the
Handicapped and Special Groups
*Arts and Crafts for Physically and
Mentally Disabled*
by Elaine and Loren Gould
Springfield Illinois: Charles C. Thomas
Publishers, 1978.
An extensive presentation of the
implementation of craft programs for the
disabled institutionalized patient. It
describes planning, coordinating,
motivating and utilizing patients,
available space, time allocation,
equipment, staff, personnel, and
volunteers with detailed craft project
descriptions.

Pastimes for the Patient, Revised Edition
by Marguerite Ickis
New York: A.S. Barnes and Co., Inc.,
1966.
This text contains chapters on nature
crafts such as plants, terrariums, bird
crafts, chip carving, leather, drawing and
painting, weaving and fibers, and music
as well as others.

*Crafts for the Very Disabled and
Handicapped*
by Jane G. Kay
Springfield, Illinois: Charles C. Thomas,
Publishers, 1977.
Many inexpensive and simple crafts.
Decorations for both Jewish and
Christian holidays.

Kits for Kids
by Nancy Towner Butterworth and Laura
Peabody Broad
New York: St. Martin's Press, 1980.
Simple crafts, easy to read, projects and
gifts to make by children ages 3 years and
up. Excellent index of crafts by type, by
skill level and various group settings.

*Accident Prevention Manual: For the
Training Programs*
edited by Merle E. Strong
Madison, Wisconsin: American Technical
Society, 1975.
OSHA laws, safety inspections, reporting
accidents.

*How to Build Special Furniture and
Equipment for Handicapped Children*
by Ruth B. Hoffmann
Springfield, Illinois: Charles C. Thomas,
Publisher, 1970.
Mostly about wood products such as
standing boards, tables, chair equipment,
creepers, etc.

*Easy-to-Make-Aids for Your Handicapped
Child*
by Don Caston
Englewood Cliffs, New Jersey: Prentice-
Hall Inc., 1981.
From measuring child, to buying supplies
and construction for 40 projects.

Safety Manual: Ceramics
by AMACO
Indianapolis, Indiana: American Art
Clay Co., Inc., 1988.
Covers all aspects of hazards in ceramics
from clay, to glazes, to firing to kiln wash.
AMACO brand specific.

Appendix III

▼

Completed Activity Analysis

Following is a sample completed activity analysis. The therapist can refer to it to determine what might be an appropriate response. On this activity analysis form, all performance components will be completed although in actual practice a therapist might choose to do only one or two.

Activity Analysis

I. Name of activity—*Leather belt*

II. Patient information (for a hypothetical patient)

    A. Diagnosis—*Drug addiction to alcohol with multiple uses of many other illegal drugs; peripheral neuropathy with weakness in all extremities.*

    B. Age—*23*

    C. Sex—*Male*

    D. Cultural identification—*Hispanic*

    E. Occupation—*Unskilled day laborer*

    F. Educational level—*Tenth grade*

    G. Family situation—*Unmarried; estranged from parents, brothers and sisters due to alcohol problem.*

III. Treatment goal for which activity is intended—*To build self-esteem through completion of an attractive object valued in the Hispanic culture.*

IV. Treatment setting requirements—*Occupational therapy clinic in a county drug and alcohol treatment center.*

    A. Size of room—*30ft. by 15ft. with a 6ft. by 6ft. storage room for supplies.*

B. Working space per person—*30sq.ft. of floor space; 9sq.ft. of table surface.*

C. Furniture arrangement (use diagram if necessary)—*The clinic has four 8ft. by 3ft. work tables in a U-shaped arrangement.*

D. Lighting requirements—*Normal indoor fluorescent lighting.*

E. Equipment and appliances—*N/A.*

F. Ventilation and temperature—*The occupational therapy clinic has a special vent and filter system to comply with institutional safety standards.*

V. Materials and tools needed; amount and cost of each—*Prices here are figured according to the 1991 institutional discount given to occupational therapy clinics.*

One 36in. x 1 1/4in. 8oz. leather belt strip—$4.00.

One 4in. x 3 1/2in. rectangle of 5oz. weight tooling leather—.50
   3ft. of leather lace.

Rectangular buckle blank for western-style buckle—$1.80.

Rotary punch—$30.00.

1in. oblong slotting punch—$9.00.

3-prong thonging chisel—$2.00.

Rawhide mallet—$14.00.

Swivel knife—$8.00.

Masonite tooling board—$3.00.

Skiver—$2.00.

Two pairs of rivets—10 cents.

Snap setter—$6.00.

Lacing needles—10 cents.

Belt design template—$2.00.

Tracing modeler—$3.00.

Edge creaser—$4.00.

Leather scissors—$18.00.

Utility knife—$4.00.

Stamping Tools

Background tool—$2.80.

Beveler—$2.50.

Pear shader—$2.50.

Seeder—$2.30.

Mink oil finish—$3.00.

Sponge applicator—50 cents.

VI. Presession preparation—*Purchase materials. Cut belt strip from cowhide back.*

A. By whom—*Certified occupational therapy assistant (COTA).*

B. Steps in preparation—*2.*

C. Time required—*Purchasing by telephone, 3min., with*

3-day wait for delivery. One-quarter hour to cut leather into belt strips.

VII. Placement of tools and materials, (eg, in cupboard, on table)—*In cupboard. Patient must get his own materials and tools as directed by the therapist.*

VIII. Steps in craft activity (number in order and describe each step including time required)

1. *Measure waist and mark leather length. (2min.)*
2. *Cut leather to correct length and shape end. Punch holes. Skive at fold. (15min.)*
3. *Cut two leather rectangles to fit buckle and cut slot for belt keeper and hole for prong. (10min.)*
4. *Wet leather with damp sponge and wait until it returns to natural color. (5min.)*
5. *Place template on leather.*
6. *Use tracing modeler to imprint leather. (15min.)*
7. *Mark belt edge with edge creaser. (5min.)*

End of session one and clean-up

8. *Allow leather to dry overnight.*
9. *Cut outline of design with swivel knife. (10min.)*
10. *Dampen leather with sponge. (1min.)*
11. *Bevel lines of design. (10min.)*
12. *Use background tool. (10min.)*
13. *Use pear shader and modeling spoon to contour leather. (15min.)*
14. *Use seeder to emphasize design. (5min.)*

End of session two and clean-up

15. *Cut slots for lacing buckle. (5min.)*
16. *Apply mink oil to grain side of belt strip and both sides of buckle. (15min.)*
17. *Allow to dry.*

End of session four and clean-up

18. *Lace buckle together using double cordovan lacing. (1 hour)*
19. *Rivet buckle to belt. (10min.)*

End of session four and clean-up

IX. Method of instruction, (eg, demonstration, verbal directions, audio or visual aid)—*Verbal directions as well as demonstration on scraps when necessary.*

X. Opportunities for grading activity
    A. Simpler to more complex—*(1) Patient can develop own design and trace it on; (2) can use greater variety of stamping tools.*
    B. Complex to simpler—*(1) Use picture stamps or alphabet letters; (2) a simple belt buckle rather than a leatherlaced buckle.*

XI. Precautions (eg, balance/gait or suicidal risk)—*Patient could still have "the shakes." Using sharp tools could be dangerous.*

XII. Sensory motor aspects
    A. Sensory awareness/processing
        1. Does the craft stimulate the visual system? How?
          Yes, the patient will see many designs before choosing.
        2. Is the auditory system stimulated by this craft? How?
          Yes, by the mallet and stamping tools.
        3. Does the craft process stimulate the olfactory system? How?
          Yes, by the leather and mink oil.
        4. Does the gustatory system receive stimulation? How?
          N/A.
        5. What tactile involvement is required?
          The wetness of the leather, smoothness of the leather and cold hardness of the tools.
        6. Is proprioception/kinesthesia/orientation of the body in space involved in this activity? How?
          Yes, the patient needs to know how high to raise his arm to use the mallet. There is proprioceptive input into the joints during pushing and pulling on the tools during hammering. There is much arm/shoulder movement.
        7. Does the craft involve vestibular/equilibrium stimulation? How?
          There is very little of this kind of stimulation as most of the time the patient is sitting.
        8. Is temperature awareness necessary in order to do this activity? When?
          Only when getting water from the faucet.
    B. Sensory perceptual skills
        1. Is stereognosis, knowing by feel, necessary during this process? When?
          The activity can be done without it.
        2. Is awareness of body scheme or position of the body in space essential in this activity? When?
          Yes, when measuring the waist size for the length of the belt.
        3. Does the patient need to discriminate the right from the left side in this craft? When?

Yes, in order to properly lace and attach the buckle with the design right side up and the belt lapping from the left to the right side.

4. Is it necessary to be able to distinguish whether forms, shapes and spaces are the same? When?
   Yes, in choosing the right size of stamping tools and in choosing the correct size of slots for the size of needle to be used.

5. Will it be necessary for the patient to distinguish a figure or object from its background?
   Yes, lacing requires this skill. Choosing rivets requires selecting one from a container. Tooling also requires focusing on the object apart from the background.

6. Will the patient be required to use depth perception to do this task? Explain.
   Yes, depth perception is necessary to aim and judge the force needed in hammering, and in pressing in the design.

XIII. Neuromuscular

A. Which joint movements are involved? (eg, flexion, extension, abduction, adduction)

1. *Measuring—Finger flexion, thumb opposition, wrist flexion and extension; elbow flexion and extension; shoulder internal and external rotation, flexion, extension and scapular retraction.*

2. *Cutting leather—Cylindrical grasp, elbow flexion and extension, should extension. Punching holes—cylindrical grasp.*

3. *Cutting and slotting leather—Cylindrical grasp, wrist radial extension, elbow flexion and extension.*

4. *Wetting leather—Tip prehension, cylindrical grasp, elbow flexion and extension, should horizontal abduction.*

5. *Placing templates—Finger extensors and flexors.*

6. *Imprinting leather and edge creasing—Finger flexion and extension, thumb opposition, wrist flexion and extension; elbow flexion and extension.*

7. *Using swivel knife—Modified 3-jaw chuck grasp, wrist radial and ulnar deviation.*

8. *Dampening leather—Thumb adduction, finger flexion and extension, wrist and elbow flexion and extension, shoulder horizontal abduction and adduction.*

9. *Beveling—Finger and thumb-tip prehension, cylindrical grasp, wrist flexion and extension, forearm supination and pronation, elbow flexion and extension.*

10. *Background—Finger and thumb-tip prehension, cylindrical grasp, wrist flexion and extension, forearm supination and pronation, elbow flexion and extension.*

11. *Pear shader and modeling spoon—Finger and thumb-tip prehension, cylindrical grasp, wrist flexion and extension, forearm supination and pronation, elbow flexion and extension.*

12. *Seeder—Finger and thumb-tip prehension, cylindrical grasp, wrist flexion and extension, forearm supination and pronation, elbow flexion and extension.*

13. *Slot on buckle—Finger and thumb-tip prehension, cylindrical grasp, wrist flexion and extension, forearm supination and pronation, elbow flexion and extension.*

14. *Apply mink oil—Same as #9.*

15. *Lace buckle—Tip prehension and 3-jaw chuck, wrist flexion and extension, forearm supination and pronation; elbow flexion and extension.*

16. *Riveting—Tip prehension, cylindrical grasp, wrist flexion and extension, forearm pronation and supination, elbow flexion and extension.*

B. Are movements passive or active?—*Mostly active; a few passive motions due to gravity.*

C. Which of the muscle groups are involved?—*Flexors, extensors of fingers 1–5, wrist, elbow and shoulder; thumb opposition; supinators/pronators of forearm; external and internal rotators of shoulder.*

D. How much range of motion is necessary? (eg, full, limited, moderate)—*Full for hand, wrist and elbow; moderate for shoulder.*

E. Is muscle tone limiting completion of task? (eg, spasticity, flaccidity)—*May be some muscle weakness and incoordination.*

F. Is coordination fine or gross?—*Both fine and gross.*

G. How will the patient be positioned? (eg, seated, standing, lying down)—*Seated.*

H. How much endurance and strength are required in each position?—*One-hour sitting tolerance required; 15 to 25 pounds grip strength for the tools.*

I. Is an assistive device necessary?—*N/A.*

XIV. Cognition

A. Orientation (is each of the below necessary? Why?)

1. Time—*Yes, to arrive at occupational therapy on time.*

2. Place—*Yes, to know how to find occupational therapy clinic.*

3. Person—*Yes, to know why he can benefit from this activity.*

B. Attention span; longest time period required for concentration on one step—*1 hour.*

C. Memory

   1. Short-term memory requirements (10sec.) to 10min.)—*Necessary to follow oral instructions.*

   2. Recent memory requirements (hours, days, months)—*Necessary to remember where he stopped on previous day.*

   3. Long-term memory requirements (years to remote past)—*Not necessary.*

D. Comprehension level (use either age- or grade-level performance expectations)—*Sixth grade.*

E. Judgment

   1. Need for formulating an opinion—*N/A.*

   2. Need to make comparisons—*Yes, in choosing designs and finish.*

   3. Need for socially appropriate expression of opinions or responses—*Only if other patients work nearby.*

   4. Need for impulse control—*Must go step by step or risk making a mistake.*

XV. Psychosocial

A. Opportunities for testing reality of patient's own perceptions/beliefs (eg, is my behavior/perception/belief normal?)—*Yes, if patient asks for therapist's evaluation of his performance and craftsmanship, it could validate or invalidate self-perception. Patient will receive direct feedback from the efficacy of his work to test his own perceptions.*

B. Opportunities for affective expression

   1. Hostility/aggression (eg, motion such as hammering, tearing, piercing)—*Yes, hammering, pressing with spoon, cutting.*

   2. Sadness (eg, slow movements)—*Wiping can be slow and rhythmical.*

   3. Happiness (eg, pride, hope, laughter)—*Can express ethnic pride through choice of design, through completion of an esthetically pleasing item.*

   4. Loving (eg, stroking, holding)—*Wiping on water and oil.*

C. Opportunities for creative expression

   1. Ideas—*Choosing the design stimulates idea formation.*

   2. Planning—*See #5.*

   3. Inventiveness—*When grading up, this could apply.*

   4. Curiosity—*Patient could ask questions about leather tanning, preparation and alternative uses.*

     5. Use of color, shape, design—*There are opportunities to choose template pattern and colors for design if he likes.*

   D. Interpersonal opportunities

     1. Needing to cooperate with

      a. the therapist—*must cooperate with time schedule of therapist and use tools safely.*

      b. another patient—*N/A.*

      c. the group—*N/A.*

     2. Sharing tools—*Yes, other patients could need leather tools at the same time.*

     3. Increasing self-esteem—*Yes, patient may be praised by other patients and therapist on work.*

     4. Developing leadership—*This could lead to patient being able to instruct other patients on a similar project.*

XVI. Opportunities for practicing work-related skills

   A. Taking instruction—*Must take instruction from therapist.*

   B. Accepting authority—*Must accept authority of therapist.*

   C. Being able to adapt—*If design is not exactly what he wants he will need to adapt it.*

   D. Setting goals—*Steps can be planned out with patient at first session.*

   E. Planning independently/cooperatively—*He can plan independently if capable of it.*

   F. Performing independently/cooperatively—*His performance will be independent.*

   G. Showing stress management/coping skills—*If his time planning is off he may need to manage stress related to time allowed in occupational therapy clinic before cleaning up.*

   H. Demonstrating body mechanics—*Awareness of or instruction in body mechanics may be required in bending over the table to wet the leather, imprint the leather, use the edge creaser, cut and tool the design and apply the finish.*

   I. Timing/waiting—*Need to wait two times for leather to dry.*

   J. Counting—*Need to measure length; count holes to punch.*

   K. Making decisions—*Can decide on design, color, buckle design.*

   L. Evaluating self—*Can evaluate his performance outcome against initial plans and the actual belt against the clinic sample belt.*

Index

Accountability, 28-29
Activities, 23-25
Activities of Daily Living Evaluation, 14,
  64, 65
Activity analysis
  explanation of, 21
  importance of, 21-22
  methods of, 22
Activity analysis form
  development of, 22
  sample of completed, 197-204
Activity Laboratory, 159
Advance Games, 151
Aides, 29
Allen Cognitive Level Test, 11, 48, 54
Androes, Dreyfus and Bloesch Diagnostic
  Occupational Therapy Test Battery,
  92
Art therapy, 157-158
Assessments
  for ceramics, 92
  for computer art, 151
  for cooking, 138-139
  for copper tooling and metal crafts, 72
  for drawing and painting, 158-160
  for fiber crafts, 113-114
  for leatherwork, 48-49
  for mosaics, 81-83
  for needlework, 64-65
  for paper crafts, 124
  for woodworking, 33, 35
Azima Battery, 92, 159

Barris, R., 21-22
Bay Area Functional Performance
  Evaluation, 160
BH Battery, 83, 160
Biomechanical frame of reference, 12-13
Bisque stains, 104
Blind patients
  ceramics for, 105
  cooking as activity for, 143
Boston School of Occupational Therapy, 3

Bread, salt-free, 141-142
Build-a-City assessment, 124
Build-a-Farm assessment, 35
Burn patients, 105-106

Card weaving, 112
Carolyn Owens Activity Battery, 92
Ceramics
  assessments for, 92
  bibliography for, 192
  case study in, 108-109
  glazes for, 104
  origin of, 91
  process used in, 93-94
  projects in, 94-100
  supplies for, 92-93
  therapeutic applications for, 105-107
  use of, 91-92
  use of pottery wheel for, 100-104
Certified occupational therapy assistants
  (COTAs), 29
Chasing, 75
Children. See Pediatric patients
Christiaansen, R., 21-22
Clay, 93
Clinical reasoning, 17-18
Clowning, 181
Cognitive Disabilities: Expanded Activity
  Analysis (Earhart & Allen), 11
Cognitive disabilities frame of reference,
  10-11
Coil building, 96-97
Collage, 83, 124
Comprehensive Assessment Process, 83
Comprehensive Evaluation of Basic
  Living Skills, 139
Computer art
  assessments for, 151
  background of, 149-150
  case study of, 153-154
  therapeutic applications of, 151-153
  use of, 150

Cooking
assessments for, 138-139
associations with, 138
bibliography for, 194
case study for, 144-146
origins of, 138
projects for, 139-141
therapeutic applications for,
142-144
use of, 5, 138
Copper tooling and metal crafts
bibliography for, 191
case study of, 78-79
chasing and piercing in, 75
process of, 74-75
therapeutic applications of, 76-78
tools for, 72-73, 75
types of, 72-75
use of, 71
Copy Flower House Test, 159-160
Cordero, J., 21-22
Crafts. *See also* Minor media
as fads, 169
background of use of, 4-6
benefits of, 4
ceramics, 91-110, 192
computer art, 149-155
cooking, 137-147, 194
copper tooling and metal crafts, 71-80,
191
creative media, 159-185
drawing and painting, 157-168, 194-
195
explanation of, 3
fiber crafts, 111-120, 192-193
inventors of, 5-6
leatherwork, 47-61, 190
less frequently used, 169-170
mosaics, 81-89, 191-192
needlework, 63-70, 190-191
paper crafts, 125-135, 192-193
terminology related to, 4
woodworking, 5-6, 33-45, 189-190
Crayon etching, 162
Crayon resist, 162
Crocheting, 64, 112, 117. *See also*
Needlework
Cross-stitch, 65-66

Decoupage, 124, 170-171
Descartes, René, 157
Developmental frame of reference, 11
Diagnostic Test Battery, 35, 48, 159
Disabled patients. *See* Physically
disabled patients
Discharge planning, 17

Disease, 12
Draw-a-Person Catalog for Interpretive
Analysis, 159
Drawing and painting
assessments for, 158-160
bibliography for, 194-195
case study for, 164-166
origins of, 157-158
supplies for, 160-161
techniques used in, 161-162
therapeutic applications for, 162-164
use of, 158
Dyadic interaction skills group, 4
Dysfunction
definitions of, 11, 14
disease as mechanical, 12

Eating disorders, 138, 143
Elderly patients. *See* Geriatric patients
Elizur Test of Psycho-Organicity, 160
Embossing, 72
Embroidery, 63-64. *See* also Needlework

Face painting, 179-181, 183
Fiber crafts
assessments for, 113-114
bibliography for, 192-193
case study of, 118-120
projects in, 114-116
therapeutic applications for, 117-118
types of, 111-113
use of, 113
Fidler Activity Laboratory, 124
Fidler Diagnostic Battery, 159
Finger weaving, 112
Fingerpainting, 158, 162, 176
Floor looms, 117
*Focus-Skills for Assessment and
Treatment* (American Occupational
Therapy Association) (AOTA), 9
Folded paper, 126, 128
Frame of reference
biomechanical, 12-13
cognitive disabilities, 10-11
developmental, 11
explanation of, 9-10
human occupation, 14
life-style performance, 13
neurophysiologic, 10
rehabilitation, 13-14
role acquisition, 12
Frames, stain, 171
Freud, Sigmund, 157

Galen, 6
Games, noncompetitive, 183-184

Geriatric patients
    ceramics for, 107
    computer art for, 153
    cooking as activity for, 143-144
    copper tooling and metal craft for, 77-78
    drawing and painting for, 163-164
    fiber crafts for, 117-118
    leatherwork used for, 58-59
    mosaics for, 86-87
    paper crafts for, 132
    woodworking used for, 42
Gillette's Battery, 92
Glazes, for ceramics, 104
God's Eyes, 112
Goodenough, Florence, 157
Goodenough-Harris Drawing Test, 158-159
Goodman Battery, 82-83, 92, 159
Grading, 25-26
Gremlin Hunt, 151
Gross Activity Battery, 160

Hammering, 74
Handicapped patients. See Physically disabled patients
Head injury, 151
Hierarchy of human needs, 47, 48, 138
Homemaking Evaluation, 64
House-Tree-Person test, 158, 159
Human occupation frame of reference, 14

Inkle looms, 112
Inner tube printing, 175
Instrumental Activities of Daily Living Scale, 139
Insurance reimbursement for materials, 28
Interest Checklist, 139

Jacobs Prevocational Skills Assessment, 49, 139
Jazlah, Ibn, 6

Key chains, 115-116
Kilns, pottery, 103-104
Kinetic Family Drawing, 159
Knitting, 64, 112, 117. See also Needlework
"Knots," 183
Kucharvy, Thomas, 149

Lacing, for leatherwork, 54-57
Lafayette Clinic Battery, 124
Latchook
    bibliography for, 192-193
    description of, 112-113
    difficulty of, 117
Leather
    choice of, 49
    color of, 53-54
Leatherwork
    assessments for, 48-49
    bibliography for, 190
    case study of, 59-60
    lacing used in, 54-57
    origin of, 5-6, 47
    process of, 50-51
    therapeutic applications of, 57-59
    tools for, 49-53
    use of, 47-48
Life-style performance frame of reference, 13
Linoleum prints, 174-175
Long-term goals, 17, 28
Looms, 112, 117
Loopers, 114-115

Macramé
    bibliography for, 192-193
    for boys, 117
    description of, 113
    projects using, 115-116
Magazine Picture Collage, 124
Magic, 183
Maslow, Abraham, 47
Materials
    cost of preparation of, 27-28
    use of raw vs. prepared, 27
Mattis' Dementia Rating Scale, 160
Mentally ill patients. See Psychiatric patients
Metal crafts. See Copper tooling and metal crafts
Milwaukee Evaluations of Daily Living Skills (MEDLS), 64
Mime, 181-182
Minor media
    explanation of, 169
    types of, 170-176
Monoprints, 172
Mosaics
    assessments for, 81-83
    bibliography for, 191-192
    case study of, 87-88
    origin of, 81
    therapeutic applications for, 85-87
    tools used in, 84
    treatment tools with, 83-84
    use of, 81
Murals, 83, 161

Nature printing, 124, 171-172
Needlepoint. *See* Needlework
Needlework
  assessment of, 64-65
  bibliography for, 190-191
  case study of, 68-69
  supplies for, 65-66
  therapeutic applications for, 67-68
  types of, 63-64
  use of, 64
Needs hierarchy, 47, 48, 138
Nedra Gillette Battery, 83
Nelson Clark's Clay Test, 92
Neurophysiologic frame of reference, 10
Neuropsychiatric Institute (NPI) Interest
    Checklist, 49, 64, 65, 83, 114, 139, 160
NPI Interest Checklist, 49, 64, 65, 83,
    114, 139, 160

Occupational therapy
  funding for, 27-28
  process of, 17
  programs for, 5
Occupational Therapy (Willard &
    Spackman), 4-5, 9, 158
O'Kane Diagnostic Battery for
    Psychiatry, 92, 159
Origami, 126, 128

Painting. *See also* Drawing and painting
  bibliography for, 194-195
  face, 179-181
Pantomime, 181-183
Paper crafts
  assessments for, 124
  bibliography for, 192-193
  case study of, 132-134
  materials for, 123
  origins of, 123
  therapeutic applications of, 131-132
  types of, 125-130
  use of, 124
Paper maché, 123, 125
Paper weaving, 126-128
Parachute games, 183
Pasta salad, 140-141
Pediatric patients
  ceramics for, 106-107
  computer art for, 153
  cooking as activity for, 143
  copper tooling and metal craft for, 77
  drawing and painting for, 163
  fiber crafts for, 117
  leatherwork used for, 58
  mosaics for, 86
  needlework for, 67-68

papercrafts for, 131-132
  woodworking used for, 41-42
Perkins Tile Task, 83
Physically disabled patients
  bibliography for, 195-196
  ceramics for, 105-106
  clowning as outlet for, 181
  computer art for, 151-152
  cooking as activity for, 142
  copper tooling and metal craft for, 76
  drawing and painting for, 162-163
  fiber crafts for, 117
  leatherwork for, 57-58
  mosaics for, 85-86
  needlework for, 67
  paper crafts for, 131
  woodworking for, 39-40
Piercing, 75
Pilgrim stool, 36, 38
Piñatas, 128-130
Pinch pots, 94-95
Pinel, Phillipe, 6
Planishing, 74
Pottery wheel, 100-103
Prescribing Occupational Therapy
    (Dunton), 5
Principles of Occupational Therapy
    (Willard & Spackman), 4-5
Printing
  description of, 172-173, 195
  inner tube, 175
  linoleum, 174-175
  nature, 124, 171-172
  vegetable, 175-176
  woodblock, 172
Printing presses, 172-173
Project Magic, 183
Psychiatric patients
  computer art for, 152-153
  cooking as activity for, 142-143
  copper tooling and metal craft for,
      76-77
  drawing and painting for, 163
  fiber crafts for, 117
  leatherwork used for, 58
  mosaics for, 86
  needlework used for, 67
  paper crafts for, 131
  woodworking used for, 41

Rationale. *See also* Clinical reasoning
  benefits of development of, 19
  as step in treatment planning, 17-18
Rehabilitation
  crafts as treatment media for, 4
  use of crafts for, 4

Rehabilitation frame of reference, 13-14
Role acquisition frame of reference, 12
Rush, Benjamin, 6

Salt-free wheat bread, 141-142
Scoreable Self-Care Evaluation, 139
Sculpture
    ceramic, 98
    paper, 128-130
Serigraphy, 172
Sewing, 63. *See also* Needlework
Shoemyen Diagnostic Test Battery, 82,
    92
Silk screen, 172-174
Skinner, B. F., 149
Slab building, 95-96
Slice of Life game, 183-184
Slip casting, 98-99
Sobriety game, 184
Software programs, 150, 151
Stain frames, 171
Stick weaving, 112
Street Survival Skills Questionnaire, 139
Strip weaving, 112
Studies in Invalid Occupation (Tracy),
    6-7
Stuffed celery, 140
Supplies
    for ceramics, 92-93
    for drawing and painting, 160-161
    for mosaics, 84
    for needlework, 65-66

Task group, 4
Textbooks, view of crafts in, 4-7, 169
Therapeutic applications
    for ceramics, 105-107
    for clowning, 181
    for computer art, 151-153
    for cooking, 142-144
    for copper tooling and metal craft,
        76-78
    for drawing and painting, 162-164
    for fiber crafts, 117-118

for leatherwork, 57-59
    for mime, 182
    for mosaics, 85-87
    for needlework, 67-68
    for paper crafts, 131-132
    for woodworking, 39-42
Three-legged stool, 36, 37
Tiled Trivet Assessment, 83
Tooling, 72
Tools
    for copper tooling and metal crafts,
        72-73, 75
    for leatherwork, 49-53
    for mosaics, 84
    for woodworking, 35-36
Treatment planning approaches, 17
Typesetting, 172

Underglazes, 104
Ungame, 183-184

Vegetable printing, 175-176
Vendors list, 187-188
Visual Organization software, 151
Volunteers, 29

Weaving
    bibliography for, 192-193
    description of, 111-112
    with paper, 126-128
Woodblock printing, 172
Woodburning, 42
Woodcarving, 38-39
Woodworking
    assessments for, 33, 35
    bibliography for, 189-190
    case study of, 42-44
    equipment for, 35-36
    origins of, 5-6
    projects for, 36-38
    therapeutic applications for, 39-42
    tools for, 35-36
    use of, 33